DATE			

BRAIN SURGEON

BRAIN SURGEON

AN INTIMATE VIEW
OF HIS WORLD

by
Lawrence Shainberg

J. B. LIPPINCOTT COMPANY · PHILADELPHIA AND NEW YORK

For my parents

U.S. Library of Congress Cataloging in Publication Data

Shainberg, Lawrence, birth date.
  Brain surgeon.

  1. Brain—Surgery—Cases, clinical reports,
statistics. I. Title.
RD594.S5   617'.481   79-1038
ISBN-0-397-01310-8

CONTENTS

Author's Note

The ground rules for this book were set by the principal surgeons involved: no real names would be used, not even the hospital's or the city in which it is located. Since authenticity and immediacy are functions of narrative rather than literal identity, and all events here portrayed happened in reality, the story has been served, not diminished, by the rules. The great limitation they place upon me is that I cannot acknowledge my principal collaborators, the surgeons and patients who lived these events and imprinted them in my mind. They know who they are, and they know too that without their help these pages would not exist.

Endless gratitude as well to others. My brother, David Shainberg, not only encouraged me and tempered my enthusiasms but occupied a large part of the middle ground between my sensibility and the neurosurgeons'. Those who read this book will know what it meant to have the instruction and assistance of a man who is trained in neurology and psychiatry but restricted by neither, as much aware of the material world as the void from which it derives, and staunch in his refusal to choose sides in the argument between them.

Thanks, too, to Gloria and Peter Watts for reading and solace at a time when both were more than normally required. To Rudy Wurlitzer, Irini Spanidou, Elizabeth Aldrich, and Steven Shainberg for rigorous, impolite criticism. To my editor, Beatrice Rosenfeld, whose belief in this project often dwarfed my own. And finally, to Min Pai and my fellow students at the Wellspring Zendo, whose support was constant, energizing, and implicitly instructive with regard to this material.

It should be noted here that superscripts have been omitted from the text so as not to impede its momentum. Those who require bibliographic references will find them, keyed to the textual page numbers, in the chapter notes at the end of the book.

BRAIN SURGEON

Men ought to know that from nothing else but the brain come joys, delights, laughter and sports, and sorrows, griefs, despondency and lamentations. And by this, in an especial manner, we acquire wisdom and knowledge, and see and hear, and know what are foul and what are fair, what are bad and what good, what are sweet and what unsavoury; some we perceive by habit and some we perceive by utility . . . and by the same organ we become mad and delirious, and fears and terrors assail us, some by night and some by day, and dreams and untimely wanderings, and cares that are not suitable, and ignorance of present circumstances, desuetude and unskillfulness. All these things we endure from the brain.

—Hippocrates, *On the Sacred Disease*

The tears stream down my cheeks from my unblinking eyes. What makes me weep so? . . . Perhaps it is liquefied brain.

—Samuel Beckett, *The Unnamable*

Prologue

When I met James Brockman in January 1976, he was chief of neurosurgery at a large medical center on the East Coast. Though his department was engaged in research covering most conditions neurosurgeons treat, and he himself had become adept at all neurosurgical procedures, he was known internationally for his treatment of brain tumor in general, meningioma in particular. At sixty-three, he was two years away from compulsory retirement, and if there is any reason why he agreed to let me do this book, it might be that he had begun to think about how he would be remembered.

At the time, I was four years into a novel in which the principal subject was brain damage. It was not finished, and I had begun to think it would never be. Without completely realizing it, I had become a captive of certain mind-brain dilemmas which I had hoped to avoid, yearning after treasures that philosophers, theologians, and not a few novelists had sought for centuries. It seemed not only possible but essential to articulate precise relationships between consciousness and flesh, define categorically the distinction between animate beings and inanimate objects.

There are ways, of course, to explore the mind-brain problem intelligently. Philosophers and neurophysiologists, among others, have developed formal traditions for doing so, and there is much to learn from their arguments. But those who pursue such matters subjectively, as I did, are outside those traditions and prone to interesting delusions. The secret dream, I believe, is to concretize that which is ultimately abstract, escape thought by defining its origins, eliminate psychology by treating it as neurology. One wants to locate one's mind within one's brain, break the final barrier through a simple act of geography. No need here to elaborate this fallacy. It is amply displayed in the pages that follow. Its great irony is that it often leads one in directions opposite to those one meant to take. Attempting to demystify the mind by treating it as brain, one actually mystifies—and romanticizes—the brain. The more one seeks to order the mental process by treating it as flesh, the more elusive and "abstract" that flesh becomes.

Such intellectual disease requires drastic, nonintellectual medicine, and nothing works better, in my opinion, than the point of view one finds among a group of neurosurgeons. The more sophisticated among them may be no less interested in the mind-brain problem than philosophers or theologians, but their daily contacts with the brain itself exact from them a constant recognition of its phenomenology. What they see when they look inside the skull is stripped of almost every description and conceptualization that makes neurology romantic.

In late 1975, frustrated by the novel, I had volunteered for work on a neurology ward. It was there that I met Brockman. We had several brief discussions, seeking common ground, but it seemed to me there was none. The questions that intrigued me were not unknown to him, but he was bored with them, and those that fascinated him seemed to me reductive and mechanical, hopelessly banal.

To my surprise, however, I found that our differences made him more, not less, appealing to me, as if I'd recognized unconsciously an approach my conscious mind abhorred. Without knowing why, I sought him out, and when he invited me to watch him operate, I discovered a world which not only ignored the dilemmas that had imprisoned me but offered the perfect antidote to my romanticism. I knew then that I would write a book about neurosurgeons, preferably Brockman, and from that day on I mounted a campaign to win his cooperation.

It wasn't easy to obtain. He was no less bored by this project than he'd been by my novel, and his daily schedule left no room for extracurricular activity. After hounding him for several weeks, I began to investigate other neurosurgeons who might be more accessible. What I had not realized was that Brockman was as mercurial and impetuous as he was concrete. A month after my final entreaty, and what I'd thought to be his final rejection, I received a letter from him which referred me to a patient, Robert Simons, who, like a patient mentioned later in this book, had just recovered from his third craniotomy for brain tumor. "I've told Mr. Simons about your book," Brockman wrote, "and he is interested to discuss it with you. If he thinks it worthwhile, I might reconsider."

Robert Simons was a man who'd endured almost every curse the human brain can perpetrate, and our conversations became for me a course in brain damage and neurosurgery. Ever so often, he'd interrupt his recitation to quiz me and check the level of my response. I believe he was totally suspicious of me, convinced that because my brain was normal I would never understand him, and I don't think he was any less suspicious after we talked than he had been before. Fortunately, that was not the test I had to pass. Both he and Brockman wanted to assure themselves that I would not betray them, to acquire some confidence that my book would do no harm. On these minimal grounds, I suppose, I alleviated their fears, and several weeks later I heard from Brockman's secretary. "The Boss wants you to meet with him tomorrow on the ward."

I spent most of the next three months following him around, left for a while to visit other hospitals, returned for another month in 1977. During this time, he treated me as his student, referred patients to me almost as if I were a member of his staff. The first of those patients, as it happened, was Charlie White, whose operation would become the focus of this book. Along with Robert Simons, Brockman and Charlie educated me, and whatever merit this book contains is a gift from them to the reader.

1

Trapdoor

It may have been that Charlie White's tumor was present at his birth, but his trip to neurosurgery did not begin until the afternoon of March 25, two weeks after his thirty-first birthday, when he stood up from his desk to go to lunch and dropped to the floor with an epileptic seizure. No illness preceded the attack, no warning of any sort. He was conscious on the way to the floor, moving, as he perceived it, in slow motion, but a moment later he was comatose. For fifty seconds he felt as though his heart had stopped beating, and for three minutes his leg shook gently, as if keeping time to music. Later he remembered none of it. Fortunately, his sister, Roberta, who saw him fall, knew enough about grand mal seizures to grab a book from his desk and slip it into his mouth to keep him from biting his tongue.

Six days later, processed now by all the technology and expertise available to neurosurgeons, he came to Osler Memorial Hospital with his mother and sister, took the elevator to the ninth floor, and sat down with Dr. James Brockman, the man they called the Boss around this particular ward, to hear the news about his illness.

Since my own travels on the ward had begun the after-noon before, Charlie and I met that evening, just before he learned that his seizure had been caused by a tumor in his brain. As we'll see, our voyages through neurosurgery would define each other exactly as health and illness do and—some would say—as imagination and reality do. My function here would often seem a mockery of his, but in a sense it represented everything he'd left behind when he collapsed with his seizure: imagination, play, and freedom, all the flights and energies that we associate with what we call "the mind." It was Charlie more than anyone else who taught me that the worst effect of brain disease is the filter it inserts between its victim and his mind.

It was a cold, wet March afternoon, and for all the weak-ness in his knees, Charlie was inexplicably excited. Since his seizure, life had been intense. He saw everything, took nothing for granted. There were times when it seemed he'd never known a better emotional state, and tonight, during his meeting with the Boss, there were moments when he could not remember why he'd come.

It was fortunate for Charlie that the current state of neuroradiology permits observation of the human brain, without incision. By the time I met him, he'd had an X-ray of his cerebral tissue called a CAT-scan and an X-ray of his cerebral circulatory system called an angiogram. Both had indicated the presence of a tumor called meningioma (be-cause it grows from the brain's external membranes, the meninges) just above the motor strip on the left-hand side of his brain. Since such tumors are seldom malignant, the odds, these odds, at least, were in Charlie's favor. Still, the deadly thing about brain tumors, in contrast to tumors in other regions of the body, is that they have no room for expansion. Since the brain is surrounded by the skull, which in effect is a sheet of armor, tumors can only grow by pressing against brain tissue itself. A perfectly benign tumor—once it has attained a certain size—can in a very short time indeed cause seizures, paralysis, muteness, amnesia, or death.

Charlie had come to Brockman by the usual route. His family doctor had sent him to a neurologist, and the neurologist had ordered X-rays. When the X-rays were ready, the neurologist consulted with the radiologist and sent him back to the family doctor with the recommendation that he see a neurosurgeon.

"Who?" Charlie had said.

Fortunately for him, his doctor replied, "If it were me, I'd see a fellow named Brockman. James Brockman."

I say fortunately, because there happened to be a glut of neurosurgeons on the market. From a profession that once attracted only oddball medical students, those who weren't intimidated by meager results or high mortality rates, neurosurgery had grown into one with such cachet that often there weren't enough patients to go around. In fact, a recent study has suggested that students leaning in the direction of neurosurgery be encouraged to lean toward something else. There were 2,985 neurosurgeons (twenty-five of them women) in the United States in 1977, double the number (per capita) practicing in Canada and four times the number practicing in England. What this meant was that there were a lot of surgeons looking for patients, and no shortage of people who'd be glad to operate on Charlie. It was the luck of his draw that directed him to Brockman, who did fifty or sixty meningiomas a year, rather than another of the 2,985 who—considering themselves perfectly competent to undertake such a procedure —did but one or two.

Since Brockman was, to say the least, a busy man, six weeks to three months behind the present in his appointment schedule—and meningiomas, once they have announced themselves with seizures, do not respect appointment schedules—Charlie was seen, as such patients often were, just before evening rounds rather than during regu-

lar office hours. The meeting was short and blunt. Brockman read X-rays the way most people read newspapers.
He knew at a glance what Charlie had and what he needed,
knew that surgery was the only way, except for surrender,
that his tumor could be addressed. What was necessary
was that Charlie understand enough to choose surgery or
reject it intelligently, with at least as much free will as
remained available to him.

"What can I tell you?" Brockman said. "You've got a
tumor."

We were sitting around a conference table in a small
room behind the nurses' station, the Boss and I, with two
residents and an intern on one side, Charlie and Roberta
and their mother on the other. The lighting in the room was
almost theatrical, a mix of overhead fluorescents, white
tile walls, and white linoleum floor. The table was white
Formica. Imprisoned by the glare, faces were spotlighted,
melodramatic and unreal.

I had not expected to be admitted to this meeting, but
Brockman had insisted that I come. "Come on," he said,
when I lingered outside the door. "I'll show you how it's
done." After a while I would come to understand that my
presence here, as in the operating room, was not, for
Brockman, without its educative value. Like many neurosurgeons, he found it best to avoid, as much as possible,
the psychology of his patients. He was not insensitive, but
he knew he would do better by a brain if he could minimize
its connections to a mind. Through me, I think, he hoped
to satisfy a certain curiosity he had always felt but never
been able sufficiently to indulge: what was it like to know
a patient on the table? He wanted me to know Charlie
White, become his friend, then watch his neurosurgery,
and he wanted to see through me how that operation
would differ from another, when the brain exposed was, as
they say, anatomy. If I was embarrassed to intrude on a
meeting such as this, the embarrassment itself was one of

the benefits Brockman derived from my presence on the ward.

Charlie was a short, stocky fellow with hyperactive eyes and a beard that mounted toward them on his cheeks. Like a lot of patients I would meet, he was more composed than his family. His mother gasped when she heard Brockman's pronouncement, and Roberta flinched as if someone had struck her, but Charlie took it straight, clear-eyed, not— it seemed to me—without a certain pride. Throughout most of the meeting, he held his mother's hand and stroked it. It's true his eyes were often downcast, but they were focused, as he would tell me later, on the Boss's hands. Aspiring novelist, English teacher by profession, addicted moviegoer, how could he resist the temptation to imagine where those hands were soon to go? "Man, every time I looked at them, I saw them in my brain." Later, he would call his illness "a trip" and "an adventure," and that too, I would discover, was not uncommon with neurosurgical patients. There were many who dissolved beneath their fear, of course, but no small number conceived of their predicament as the end of fear, a condition that made fear obsolete. By the time they got to the surgeons, they seemed to think of themselves as objects, given up to the gods (or their surrogates) for manipulation and repair. And objects, of course, though they may frighten, are not afraid themselves.

"Come here," Brockman said.

He had mounted Charlie's angiograms on a screen at one end of the room. Beautiful if studied with detachment, suggestive, in fact, of Jackson Pollock's later work, they were invented by a Portuguese neurologist named Antonio de Egas Moniz in 1929, a series of X-rays taken after radiosensitive dye, injected through a principal artery, has caused the major vessels of the brain to "light up" in contrast.* Almost alone, this technique revolutionized neurosurgery (and other specialties too), making unnecessary a great deal of what used to be called exploratory surgery. The prints it produced, which we saw now, were tangles of black on white that snaked around a central mass like the roots of an oak stretched out from its trunk. There were three prints, three different angles, and close to the top of each was the walnut-sized mistake that had pressed down into Charlie's brain and dropped him to the floor. Brockman drew a circle around it with his fountain pen.

"This is the tumor. See it? And here it is from another angle. It's just above the motor strip, growing down into what we call the falx. That's why it gave you a seizure in your leg." And then, with a flourish that was no less comic for being compassionate, he touched his own head with his fountain pen, describing a circle just behind the crown. "I'd say that the tumor is just about here."

"Damn," Charlie said, "that's just where I felt it. So I didn't imagine it after all."

"No," said Brockman, smiling. "I guess you didn't." He turned to another modern miracle, the CAT-scans. CATs—for Computerized Axial Tomography—have been around since 1973, offering surgeons and patients a painless method of examining brain tissue. Unlike angiography, which can be extremely uncomfortable, even dangerous at times, CAT-scans involve nothing more than common X-rays, no injections or discomfort, none of the heat flash that occurs when the dye rushes into the head. Patients simply lie on a table and keep their heads in a rubber collar while a huge machine moves around them, taking pictures. In fact, the CAT takes many, many pictures of narrow horizontal sections of the brain and then reassembles them by computer,

---

* Interestingly enough, Moniz won a Nobel Prize in 1949, not for his extraordinary work in radiology but for his part in the development of the now-discredited operation called prefrontal lobotomy.

eventually permitting simple Polaroid prints to be made of the tissue that interests the surgeons. It was one of these prints that Brockman presented now.

"See that? There's the tumor again!"

A chain-smoker (three packs a day), he leaned back in his chair and lobbed half a cigarette toward the wastebasket. Except in the operating room, he was almost never not smoking, and disposing of butts was a constant challenge that sometimes produced unfortunate results. The week before, according to a resident, a wastebasket employed in this fashion had burst into flames during just such an interview as this.

"Why did I get it?" Charlie said.

"No one knows why these things happen. Some people think they're viral, and some say they're genetic. For all we know, even stress can bring them on."

"Worry? Could worry do it? Lately I've had a lot of things on my mind."

The Boss laughed. "I doubt that, but what the hell, your guess is as good as mine."

He lit another cigarette, waiting for questions he knew would come. At the end of the table, the intern was eating a candy bar, rustling the paper, and Brockman glared at him until he stuffed it in his pocket.

"What's the danger?" Charlie said.

"If we go for it?" Brockman got up and went to the angiogram again. "See this large vein?" He indicated a curving line beneath the tumor. "If the tumor is blocking this vein, we can take it all. If not, we'll have to leave a piece inside." (What he was pointing to was not, in fact, a vein at all but a large draining vessel called the sagittal sinus, which is sometimes referred to as a vein for purposes of simplification. When a meningioma blocks this vessel entirely, the brain usually develops ancillary drainage to replace it, and the danger of transecting it, during surgery, is diminished. It is when the sagittal sinus is partially blocked, and still the only means of drainage, that the risks increase.)

Mrs. White, who had neither spoken nor raised her eyes since the interview began, put her first question now, in a whisper that could barely be heard. "Speech," she said. "What about speech?"

"No need to worry about that." Once again Brockman touched his own head, this time just above the left ear. "Speech is way up here. There may be some weakness in his tongue, a little slurring of words, but it won't last long."

"His leg?"

"That's a danger. We can't pretend it isn't. If he has any deficit, that's where it will be."

He was, as we see, not much for euphemism. Interviews like this could sometimes become shock therapy, but brutal as he could sound to innocents like me, patients would tell you he refreshed them. Most of them, it seemed, had heard nothing but uncertainty since their illnesses began. Seizures and headaches, confusion, ringing in the ears—neurological symptoms are often vague and transient, and more than any others, they make physicians insecure. The temptation to wait and think it over is sometimes irresistible. Imagine what it meant, after four or five such inconclusions, to meet a man who thrived on decisions and had no fear of the risks his decisions imposed.

Now it was Roberta's turn. As older sister, she was trying to keep things in order, but it was clear that she was much worse off than Charlie. "What happens if you don't operate?"

Brockman was so used to this question that his answer was almost eloquent. For all his toughness, he had particular style in moments like this, a spontaneity on the one hand and a loathing for cant on the other that could defuse the terror about to surface. Others sat with patients

longer or displayed more visible compassion, but he got to
the bottom line so fast that no room was left for anticipation or imagination or, for that matter, thought—where
the worst of the fear resided.

"Sooner or later it will kill him."

Meetings like this followed more or less the same pattern—there weren't, after all, that many questions to ask
—and at this point they usually ground to a halt. It seemed
as if we stood together on a cliff, looking over the edge.
The intern nibbled at his candy bar again, and Benny Richmond, the chief resident, on the Boss's right, played with
the tuning fork he used to test patients for tumors of the
acoustic nerves. The other resident sat with his eyes closed
as if sound asleep. Brockman, however, did not look away.
He was watching Mrs. White, and now he reached and took
her hand.

"What do you want to know?"

"If it were you," she said, "what would you do?"

"Me? Hell, I'd have it out. But I'm a surgeon. You can't
listen to me. This is something you've got to decide for
yourselves."

The next question, though less serious, was a lot more
awkward. Everyone asked it, stumbling and embarrassed,
and everyone took the answer badly.

"What sort of incision do you make?"

"Oh, that's not a problem," he said. He indicated a U-
shaped line on his head, a horseshoe that began behind his
ear and ended in front of it and reached the midline at its
apex. "We make a cut here, then another here, then we
make a sort of flap in the scalp and a trapdoor through the
skull. Very simple procedure."

"Trapdoor" was vintage Brockman, pure inspiration. He
had gotten the idea somewhere that it put his patients at
their ease. Guaranteed, it was, every time, to turn them as
pale as they'd be when they came out of surgery. What he
was describing is called craniotomy, which is to say, the

opening of the skull. Of all stages in neurosurgery it is probably the least dangerous, but it is also the most shocking, the supreme violation of identity. He knew this, of course, but as a surgeon he saw the body in rather a different light from his patients or their families. What was violation to them was merely entry to him, and brilliant entry at that. Hell, they were proud of their flaps around here!

Mrs. White began to sob, but he took her hand again. "Come on, come on. It's not as bad as that. Think about it for a while and let me know what you decide."

"Why should we think about it?" Charlie said. "It's my decision and I want it out. I'd always know it's there. Never forget it. I want it out."

In all the time I was at the hospital, I saw only one patient refuse his operation, and he eventually had it done somewhere else. Avoidance of death at any cost is one of the things we take for granted in this culture, and neurosurgery is a great celebration of this endeavor. I knew I'd choose as Charlie had, if I were in his place, but after hanging around the operating room a bit, the decision became arguable, to say the least. In fact, there is nothing like neurosurgery for bringing cosmic views of death to mind, making you weigh your fear of death against the cost of fending it off. "Timely death," as Pliny the Elder called it, can seem as much like a gift as a punishment, and it may be well, as we begin this journey, to keep Pliny's words in mind: "I do not indeed hold that life ought to be so prized that by any and every means it should be prolonged. You holding this view, whoever you are, will nonetheless die . . . of all the blessings given man by Nature, none is greater than a timely death."

As it happened, Charlie's commitment was not only easy but enthusiastic. I never saw one like it again. Brockman suggested several times that he sleep on it, talk it over with his family and friends, but each time he shook his head. "I want it out. I don't want it growing in my head. When can you do it?"

Finally the Boss shrugged and turned to Benny. "You heard the man, Benny. When can we do it?"

Richmond took a notebook from his pocket and scanned the weekly schedule. "Next week looks good. How about Thursday?"

"How about next Thursday?" Brockman repeated.

Charlie leaned back in his chair. His eyes were inspired, frenetic, crazy with luminosity. It was clear that whatever he may have registered in one part of his brain about this foreign presence in another, some parts had come to terms with it.

"Dynamite!" he cried.

"All right, great," said Brockman. "Come back on Sunday and we'll get you a bed. It will take some time to get you ready."

They stood and shook hands, and then Charlie and his family left the room together.

Brockman had two more patients to see before evening rounds began, but he took a moment to investigate my state of mind. Had the meeting distressed me? When I admitted that it had, he laughed aloud and pointed at me with the same pen he had used to outline Charlie's tumor on his own head. "You'll get used to it. It's nothing. We play God every day."

It was an old cliché, and he was, of course, making fun of it. What was odd, and a little frightening, was that for a moment it seemed not excessively grandiose. One man was stalked by timely death and another had set out to stop his clock.

Brockman, as we'll see, did his best to keep this part of his work in perspective, but it was seductive. For obvious reasons, the patients liked to believe him omnipotent, and it isn't easy to play that role if you don't believe in it yourself. As Brockman put it once, when someone attacked him for confusing himself with God, "Who do you want messing around in your brain—someone who thinks he's a plumber?"

2

The Perfect Tension

Brockman dressed as he had in college, chinos or gray-flannel pants—both tapered and cuffed, with that small belt at the back that was popular once in Ivy League schools—button-down collar, and striped tie, the last often tucked into his shirt so it wouldn't get in the way when he leaned to examine patients. On the outer side of each upper arm he had a small tattoo of geometrical design, and for years he'd had his hair cut every Friday morning at the same time by the same barber into the same right-angled crew cut he had worn since high school. Once he had been a good lightweight boxer in the army, and even now—at sixty-three years—his body looked capable of three or four rounds against a man twenty years younger. He ran two miles every morning, did fifty pushups and fifty situps, jumped rope for ten minutes in his living room. "Narcissism," he explained. "I don't like being sixty-three." He was the first man I had met in fifteen years who kept his keys on the gold-link affair that hooks onto the belt loop and curls across the thigh to the pants pocket—what we used to call a key chain.

His blue eyes were astonishing in their brightness, their

mix of restlessness and concentration—a reflection of his character, as well. He was present when necessary, but when attention gave way to impatience, he terminated meetings with no transition, no nod in the direction of formality. "All right, get out of here." His residents would tell you they had chosen their appointments here over others that offered equal advantage because he had enchanted them with his honesty. No doubt there were some, now working elsewhere, who would call that honesty rudeness, but these, his disciples, when they had come for interviews and found him barefoot, his feet on the desk, had discovered the home they thought they needed to develop the skills they hoped, above all, would someday equal his. Barefoot or not, of course, he would not have drawn them to his office if it weren't for his reputation. "I asked four of my professors for advice," one recalled, "and each one said, 'If Brockman will take you, train with him.' "

To say the least, Brockman's work was a family tradition. Both his grandfather and father had been, like him, not just surgeons but professors of surgery, chiefs of their departments in the large southern city where he was born and where, even now, the family remained a ubiquitous medical presence. One of his uncles was a professor of gynecology, another of cardiology, one cousin was dean of the medical school, and three others were on its teaching staff. His own son, an aspiring painter who hated the sight of blood, would break the tradition; he had never seen his father operate, never felt an inclination toward medicine.

In contrast, Brockman had made rounds with his father at the age of seven, and his earliest memories of the breakfast table revolved around discussions of the gallbladder or lung to be removed that afternoon. At moments of rebellion he had imagined himself an architect, but in fact it was accepted early, by him and others, that he would be a doctor, if not necessarily a surgeon. There was no inclination toward surgery until he began operating on dogs in medical school, but one week in the lab—one week of the immediacy and concreteness and the intimacy one felt when fingertips moved beyond skin—took care of that. Like his father and grandfather and those of his colleagues who shared his demonic infatuation, he was addicted to the work from the moment he opened flesh.

But at first, under the heading of flesh, the brain was not included. Indeed, neurosurgery had interested him so little that when the army offered him a choice between a battalion aid station at the front and a neurosurgical position at the base, he chose the former. Had his father been less influential—both in his son's life and in the American medical establishment—Brockman might be a chest surgeon today, but it so happened that the old man was the type who'd not only reprimand his son for such stupidity, but get on the phone to the Surgeon General in Washington. "Don't listen to the little bastard," he said. "Give him neurosurgery." The army obeyed his command, and Brockman obeyed the army's, and after two months of working on the brain, Brockman was hooked. He never looked back.

Brockman's father was neither the first nor the last to use the the adjective "little" with reference to him. He was five-foot-three, and there were those, even among his friends, who considered his lack of height to be the engine that drove his life. It wasn't difficult to attribute his ambition and success to a little-man complex that had found its perfect consummation. What was good to know was that he not only saw it that way himself but acknowledged it with enthusiasm. No one was better than he at picking himself apart, and as he saw it, his size had served him well. "I was a little kid, always fighting bigger kids. Maybe I've never stopped. It wouldn't take much imagination to lay my whole career on the need to be bigger than I am."

The army, of course, was a good place to begin working on the brain: lots of head wounds during wartime, lots of brain damage. In fact, much of the pioneer work on brain damage (like Kurt Goldstein's and A. R. Luria's) was done on war wounds. But even without these fillips, Brockman thought neurosurgery would have caught him up eventually. "There's no field as challenging, none as dangerous and risky, none that lays down such responsibility and anxiety or imposes so many life-or-death decisions. Heart surgeons may have as much anxiety, but they make only one decision. Once they begin a procedure, they have no options. For us, each decision leads to another. We can get a large part of a tumor, then find ourselves looking at more. Do I go for the whole thing? Is that piece gonna hurt him if I leave it there? Am I gonna hurt him by getting it? Often, you see, we don't know what that piece is attached to. Not too long ago I went after the last part of an acoustic tumor and split open a basilar artery. The guy never recovered. It's not like that in heart, certainly not in general. General surgeons deal with muscle. We deal with brain. The dysfunctions we can produce are horrible."

That was one way to look at it, from the outside in. The other was from the inside, the particular inclination and idiosyncrasy that sent one off in this direction. "There are two reasons you can choose to be a neurosurgeon. Talk to my colleagues and you'll find they were either interested in the neural sciences or attracted by surgery itself, the management of power, the all-or-nothing aspect of its decisions. For me it was the latter. All the powerful figures in my childhood were surgeons. It doesn't take any great psychoanalytic insight to see what neurosurgery offered. Shit, my personality is transparent. Do you know what I do when I'm on vacation? I get on my boat and go out fishing, looking to catch a fish twice my size. What I love best is to take the boat out twenty miles and bring it back in bad weather, on instruments. If you wanted to do a textbook on the surgical personality, you'd get a head start if you began with me."

In addition to the medical atmosphere in which he'd grown up, there were other influences, equally obvious, that had shaped his personality. As a child, he had lacked nothing but happily married parents. There were four servants in the house, private schools, no brothers or sisters to compete for the attention that (by his own estimate) spoiled him hopelessly. When the divorce came, he was five years old, and among its ramifications there were two which, as he saw it, were crucial to his life. Since his mother ("Really beautiful," he said, "and really promiscuous") moved away, he and his father were left alone with a rivalry that would enrage and nourish them both as long as they lived. "An interesting relationship," Brockman called it in remarkable understatement, and it was amplified—when the son's prestige began to equal his father's—by the ethos of the medical world itself. Nothing, in fact, said more about that world than the manner in which their rivalry was consummated.

"At seventy-three," he recalled, "the old man was still operating, even though he was partially senile. He had such a reputation that, even though he was always having to be bailed out by his residents, patients begged for him. Everyone on his staff was afraid of him, and whenever they summoned the courage to talk to him about retirement, he'd have tantrums. Finally they called me about it and we worked out a plan, the only way we could figure to ease him out. I was invited to speak at the medical school, and he came to hear me talk. While he was there, the board of trustees met and—since he was a member of the board, they had to do this when he was absent—voted to strip him of his operating privileges. It was my job to break the news—after the lecture, when we were driving home. It wasn't a total wipe-out—Christ, they'd made him head of the Cancer Clinic—but he wouldn't speak to me for six months."

The second ramification of his parents' divorce was an obsession with his mother that had him, throughout high school and college, driving to New York, twelve hours each way, to visit her on weekends. Unlike the rivalry with his father, the obsession may not have been an inspiration toward neurosurgery, but it helped generate a lifelong infatuation with women that was driven, as he saw it, by the same machine that drove him in surgery. By his own admission, that machine had preoccupied and sometimes almost destroyed him. "I got married my senior year in college, but I couldn't stop fucking around. For years, it was the bane of my poor wife's existence. During my residency I fell in love with a nurse and couldn't make up my mind between her and my wife. It got me so fouled up I finally went into analysis. Luckily, I found a good doctor. He helped me a lot. I didn't give up women—God, I couldn't do that!—but at least I got it under control."

For all Brockman's psychoanalytic interpretations (remarkable in themselves, considering the organic bias of his work), there is one detail about his childhood which is tantalizing from a neurological point of view: he did not speak until he was three years old. Since the left side of the brain is dominant in the control of speech and the right in mechanical or spatial (or musical) tasks, those who speak late are often, it is postulated, developing more quickly in the right hemisphere than the left or, even more important, moving with less speed toward the left-side dominance and cerebral disequilibrium which characterizes most human adults. Not surprisingly, there is no end to the theory concerning late speech and its tendency to produce adults who excel in scientific, mathematical, or musical careers (Einstein, for instance, who did not speak until very late). Although none of these theories has been verified, Brockman's history and his mastery as a surgeon are good data to support them, wonderful stuff to think about on days (of which, for this writer, at that time, there were many) when you like to believe that all behavior originates in the brain.

When the child Brockman finally did speak, he lisped, and when he wrote, he did it backward (mirror writing). By the time he was three, his grandfather, convinced that he was retarded, had put aside five thousand dollars for his care when he was twenty-one. Even now he had left-right confusion, indicating, some think, an unusual relationship between the hemispheres. Though he could extract brain tumors, he found it difficult to dial telephone numbers, and often, when he was operating, particularly if he was using the microscope, he could not remember which hemisphere was dominant in his patient. Fortunately, he had a scar on his left thumb which, when wriggled, helped him orient himself again. You could say that he learned to trick his brain, circumvent his spatial confusion by tapping cells in other regions, approach the problem through the back door since the front was locked, and thus proceed with the business at hand.

Two days after his meeting with Charlie White, I had an appointment for an interview with Brockman at nine o'clock in the morning. It would take me some time to understand that such appointments were approximate at best, fantasies of order and continuity that never came about. Even his secretaries did not arrive before nine thirty, and though he was there some mornings by seven thirty, there were many, like this one, when he began his day elsewhere and never came to the office at all. Either way, appointments were made for nine-at-the-office with what seemed to be all good intention. He was on time when he had to be, but if the appointment wasn't urgent, there was no telling when he'd show up or if he'd show up at all.

Once I came to understand his schedule, none of this

surprised me. His days were squeezed and overstuffed, functions on the one hand of his responsibilities and on the other of his inability to say no. Like many other such people, Brockman was absolutely dependent on his secretaries, and sometimes the one who made appointments and the one who reminded him of them got their signals crossed. Even when they didn't, even when he was scheduled correctly and prompted correctly, there was always an emergency, or at least an exceptional request, and, if neither of these, a relentless distraction—a hysteria that lay behind the fantasy of order—that stalked him, never more than a step or two behind. He was generally an hour late for evening rounds, sometimes two hours late for appointments, and once he arrived at a meeting in Denver a week before it began. After a few days of following him around, I found such madness perfectly reasonable. Never mind punctuality. It seemed heroic that he made it through his day at all.

Finding the outer office door locked, I sat down to wait in a room across the hall. A typical medical waiting room with orange Leatherette furniture and magazines on the coffee table, it was, as it happened, the Visitors' Lounge that served the intensive-care units for both neurosurgery and neurology. Generally, if patients had come in during the night, you'd find their families here in the morning, waiting to talk to residents about the X-rays or the operations, waiting to see if their husbands or wives, friends, lovers, children, or parents had made it through the night.

There was no one waiting when I arrived, but a few minutes later a woman came in whose husband, as I would discover later, was being operated on that morning. She was a young black woman with short, straight hair and eyes that, like many you encountered here, shifted between anger and sadness and bewilderment and sometimes (for the lucky ones, like her) a laughter that contained them all. She had come to see her husband before he went down to the operating room, and now she would wait here until he came back. As it turned out, that wouldn't take long. When they opened him up, they found there wasn't much they could do to help him.

His name was Andrew March, and he had a kind of tumor called glioma that differed radically from Charlie White's. It was malignant, for one thing, and it grew not from the lining of the brain but from the glial cells which, along with the neurons, or nerve cells, compose the tissue of the brain. Neurons, which don't reproduce, rarely become malignant (there is a cancer called neuroblastoma, but it is extremely rare), but glial cells, which outnumber neurons by ten to one, behave in most ways like cells in other parts of the body. They can develop several different kinds of tumor, each of which will reproduce at different speeds. Though none is curable, some give their victims time and some don't. Andy March's, the fastest of all, would give him thirty-two days.

Gliomas are controversial tumors. Most everyone believed that within ten years they would be treated pharmacologically, if at all, and even now there were many who thought the only thing to do was give patients steroids— which reduce brain swelling and slow the growth of the tumor—and let them live out their days as gracefully as possible. Brockman and his department were of another school. They were known for their aggression, their willingness to enter where others had desisted. Though aware of the arguments against his position, the Boss considered it his responsibility as an academic neurosurgeon to be aggressive. Others could investigate the effects of steroids; he would take out as much tumor as he could and then explore the benefits that came when "tumor burden" was diminished. Besides, what he took was passed on to pathologists and immunologists, grown in cultures, and studied under the electron microscope. Even those who disagreed with his approach did not contest its contributions to research.

Sometimes, as I say, they'd take as much glioma as possible, but in certain cases, like Andy March's, they'd find a mass so big and so near to vital centers that any extraction was meaningless. Nothing to do then but install a shunt, or draining tube, to relieve the pressure the tumor was generating in the brain. Often, that took care of the pain and some of the side effects. What they hoped for then was that the patient would be well enough to go home. There was nothing else they could do, no reason for the patient to pay for hospitalization, and the bed was needed for others. Since this was a ward with a relatively quick turnover, the last thing they wanted was a turn for the worse that would make transfer impossible and keep the patient there indefinitely.

As it turned out, that's exactly what happened with Andy March. He had collapsed a week before while eating and, unlike Charlie, since he was unconscious, had been admitted as an emergency. Like a lot of patients I would see here, he had had symptoms he'd ignored—weakness in the leg and arm—for quite a while. By the time the tumor was found, it was enormous, and though he had regained consciousness for moments during the preceding week, he never did so after surgery. For more than a month he would lie in a coma, and his wife would sit beside his bed and watch him die.

Presently we were joined in the Visitors' Lounge by three more haggard-looking people, an elderly couple and a fat middle-aged man who turned out to be their son. They brought with them a large bucket of Kentucky Fried Chicken and, though periodically one or the other burst into tears, they spread napkins on the table and went through the meal methodically.

Their problem was the other son, who had what is called an aneurysm, more precisely a giant aneurysm. Aneurysms are swellings, deformations in blood vessels that cause them to puff out like bubbles. At this point, the wall of the vessel becomes weak and therefore susceptible to hemorrhage, and while many of those who bleed (30 percent, according to recent figures) will never make it to the hospital, most who do can be cured with surgery. In certain cases, the aneurysm grows without bleeding, causing neurological symptoms by pressing into surrounding tissue, becoming all the time more difficult to treat, swelling like a time bomb in the head. These are called giant aneurysms, and the patient whose family sat before me now had one of the biggest that Brockman or anyone on his staff had ever encountered. They had seen him two years before, when it was a peanut causing headaches; seen him last year, when it was a walnut, causing aphasia; and now he was back with a golf ball that last night had caused a seizure. Each time he'd come, they had wanted to operate, and each time the older brother, Dominic, had argued against it and prevailed. Now surgery was essential, but Dominic was still combative.

"Listen, Mama. Whatever happens, we gotta remember these aren't the only doctors in the world. We know what Victor's got. We don't need them to tell us. We gotta tell ourselves there's hospitals everywhere. Whatever they tell us, we'll get another opinion. Don't take their word for nothing!"

They were the Alfredo family. The parents were first-generation Italian immigrants, and their English was rudimentary. That was no problem for the father, who was quietly absorbed in his chicken, but the mother was locked in the struggle to express herself.

"Oh, God!" she cried. "This is-a murder. Put it in God's hands. Leave Victor to the Lord!"

Like her husband, she was into the chicken, reaching toward the bucket for another piece as soon as she was done with what she had. The coffee table was a mess, and a great pile of crumbs was accumulating at their feet. They had nodded toward Mrs. March and me when they came into the room, but if they were concerned about our presence, they gave no sign of it.

"Just remember," Dominic said, "we don't take orders from nobody. There's a doctor in California who plugs these things with glue. I read about it in the paper. Another one, in Canada, he puts a balloon in there and blows it up. No cutting, no bleeding, nothing! He puts it in the leg and slides it up to the brain! I'm gonna ask Brockman about it when I see him. Don't let them kid you, Mama. They may be smart but they don't know everything."

At nine thirty Benny Richmond unlocked the outer office door, and I followed him inside. He was pale and haggard, moving like a sleepwalker. He'd been up all night with patients (Victor among them), and he sat down now for a quick cup of coffee to prepare himself for the day ahead. In forty-five minutes he would go downstairs to assist Brockman's associate, Harvey Kellogg, in the hopeless attempt on Andy March's tumor.

Such hours were not unusual for Benny. As chief resident, he was responsible for everything that moved on the ward. The Boss and his attendings, like Kellogg, were more or less in charge of patients, but once people were admitted, the medical work—presurgical tests, for example, or postsurgical supervision—was done by residents. As a rule, Benny's day began at six thirty in the morning and ended between ten and eleven at night. He was on duty every other weekend and two nights a week, and he operated four times a week. When an interesting patient appeared, it was he who studied and researched the case to present it at conference, and often that meant hours of work in the library.

Next year, when he would be thirty-four, Benny would not be a student for the first time in twenty-six years. His postgraduate training had taken him through four years of medical school, one of internship (followed by two years in the army), one in England for neurology, and now five of neurosurgery, which requires more training than any other specialty.

It was no accident that the more sophisticated people on the staff were painfully aware of their provincialism and working hard to counteract it. The training left little time and less energy for things beyond the hospital, and even if it had, there were the other ancillary dues for it that many physicians never quite paid off: addiction to the work on the one hand, insecurity in its absence on the other. When you spent that much time with people who needed you, it could be awfully difficult to be with those who didn't. The great temptation was to hang around the hospital, extend your schedule until the time beyond it was only for sleep, and the more you succumbed to this, the less life you had outside, the more reason you had to stick around the ward. If you spent time with doctors, you could sympathize with their problem. It was uncanny how quickly I came to feel like them myself. I wasn't needed by anyone here, but after a couple of weeks around the hospital, life outside began to seem pale and diffuse by comparison. It didn't matter that the events I witnessed might be devastating. I found myself reluctant to leave, rushing back, stopping by on weekends. If I was a junky in such a short time, imagine the habit with which Benny had to contend.

Benny was a good place to start if you wanted to see how neurosurgeons came about, especially those who'd arrived at the work through what Brockman called "an interest in the neural sciences" rather than an interest in surgery. Like most such people, he was fascinated with the brain's relationship to the mind, though loath to discuss it explicitly (the mind-brain problem can generate no end of intellectual paranoia in those who choose to investigate it concretely). Benny was drawn to neurosurgery, he said, because of its "concreteness." What that meant, of course, was that its means of investigation are exquisitely direct. While neurophysiologists work with cat brains or the central nervous systems of squid, and neurologists have to content themselves with X-rays or subjective accounts of internal symptoms, neurosurgeons work straight on, every day, with living human brains. "What can I tell you?" Benny said. "I love to look at it."

The trail that brought him here had begun—in college —with a study of philosophy that narrowed to the philosophy of science, when general philosophy came to seem too abstract for his tastes, and continued—as each step in turn disappointed for the same reasons—through psychiatry and neurology. He went to medical school thinking that psychiatry would offer a "real" way to address philosophical problems, switched to neurology when he found psychiatry "a jumble of conceptualism," and when neurology proved no less frustrating, there was nowhere to go but neurosurgery. Like most people who become obsessed with the brain, he was driven by an interest in mind that yearned for nonsubjective data or, more precisely, truth beyond the mind itself. In neurosurgery, he thought he'd found it: "the perfect tension between the abstract and the concrete, a means by which the larger questions can be pursued without sinking into abstraction."

Needless to say, the larger questions got lost in the daily grind of urine bags and catheters. One does not investigate the mind while opening the skull. But when things became unbearably banal, there was always the consolation of the operating room itself. Even Benny, for all his philosophical underpinnings, had to admit that the O.R. had been, to say the least, a pleasant surprise, similar to L.S.D. or mescalin in the revelations it offered, a bit like skydiving (which he'd also tried) in its knack for stirring up adrenaline, and you'd be hard-pressed to find one among his colleagues who would argue his analogy.

While Benny drank his coffee now, the secretaries drifted in, and soon the phones and typewriters began the clamor that would continue throughout the day. By ten the daily miasma was in gear. Though it was just another busy office, the business that got transacted here made its efficiency surreal, never more than camouflage for the disasters it contained. During the first quarter hour that morning, there were calls concerning a man who'd had a seizure the night before, a young non-pregnant woman who was lactating from both breasts (a symptom frequently of pituitary tumor), and another—thirty-two years old—who had thrown herself in front of a bus an hour before and (since one of the subspecialties of the department was treatment of spinal-cord injury and head trauma) had just been admitted through the emergency ward. Near the door an obese young woman who turned out to be a medical student was raving about the epiphany she'd experienced yesterday, watching Brockman operate ("The man's an artist, there's no other way to put it!"), and behind her, taking exercise in the hall, two patients with bandaged heads stopped to listen in. When Kenneth Beck (who did most of the pediatric neurosurgery) arrived, he was informed by his secretary that one of his patients, a five-year-old, had been struck in the stomach by her brother last night. "That's fine with me," he said. "Just don't tell me she's got a headache."

Business, as I say, was certainly transacted. They were dealing, after all, with research and the education of neurosurgeons as well as with clinical patients (550 major operations the year before, almost all requiring longtime follow-up), and they were serving Brockman's career, which in certain ways had come to resemble a full-scale corporate enterprise. But every once in a while the receptionist's voice would rise above the din—"How long did you say he's been unconscious?"—and you would remember where you were. Maybe it was, as Brockman liked to

call it, "a store," but its customers were always desperate
and its commodity was life itself.

When at ten fifteen I realized that the Boss had forgotten our appointment, I asked Claire Zerilla, the department
coordinator, to page him for me. She found him in radiology, and he suggested I join him there. Often I would feel
he forgot our appointments because he was annoyed with
me for following him around, but the truth was he had
delegated memory for such things to his secretaries. Ear-
ly-morning appointments were particularly risky for that
reason, since he had been away from the office overnight.
In any event, he never apologized for missing appointments ("None of these guys," Claire said, "will ever admit
he's wrong") and frequently, when I caught up with him,
he acted as if things were running exactly according to
schedule.

"He says you should hurry," Claire said this time, as she
hung up. "He's got some stuff you ought to see."

Perhaps I might have hurried had I known my way
around the hospital, but that day was a long way off for
me. Radiology was only about a ten-minute walk from
neurosurgery, but if you weren't familiar with the building's infuriating design, the trip could take twice or three
times as long. It required negotiation of endless corridors
which, as far as I could determine, were arranged without
regard to logic. Swinging doors were everywhere but without discernible purpose, signs were incomprehensible,
elevators unmarked, mobbed, and forever delayed. There
was an old building and a new one, and the latter had four
wings off the central hub. Thus there were three banks of
elevators (one in the old building, two in the new), and five
rooms could have the same number. There was a 706, for
example, in the old building and one on each wing in the
new.

If in addition to your geographical hysteria you suffered
also from nonhabituation to the suffering that filled these

halls, travels here could seem like wanderings on a battle-field. That morning, when I stepped on the elevator, two nurses were discussing an infant who had died an hour before, and a policeman stood next to them, handcuffed to a teenager on crutches. At the third floor, the operating floor, doors opened onto a line of patients in their beds, waiting for surgery, backed up like cars in a traffic jam. In the lobby, junkies nodded out, babies howled, and most anyone who looked okay was talking to himself. To get to radiology I had to go outside, from the old building to the new, and since this took me by the parking lot, I got to see a guy who would become one of my favorites, a regular who showed up three or four times a week. He stood at the edge of the lot, waving his crutch, ordering the attendant —who was nowhere in sight—to bring up his car. "It's the silver Caddy with the TV antenna on the roof. You know the one, Mac!"

I found the Boss in the rear of the radiology department, standing in front of a large illuminated screen that was posted, at this time, with myelograms, or spinal studies, the X-rays they took when patients "presented" with back trouble. Ghostly photos they were, more disturbing than angiograms because familiar. Everyone, after all, has seen a skeleton, if only in a high-school science class, and that's all these were, shiny black sheets of film on which the spine was etched in luminous silver-gray.

"Look here," said Brockman, pointing to the screen. "This is a great-looking black girl, a model, twenty-three years old, neurotic as hell." He traced a line with his fountain pen along the lower vertebrae. "Thinks she's got a slipped disk. She doesn't. This is where it ought to be. Every time her boyfriend leaves, her back goes out. What she needs is a swimming pool, not a surgeon. I'll have a talk with her tonight."

He pressed a button and the screen rose mechanically, revealing a whole new set of myelograms, another spine, another back in agony. Nodding and muttering, he studied them intently for a moment, then once more took out his pen. "See this? That's what you call a slipped disk. This is a guy who's do-able, somebody we can help. Come on. Let's go see some angiograms."

Lighting a cigarette, he hurried down the hall, moving —as he did all day, every day—like someone who's been wound up and released and has no way to stop. He wore a knee-length white jacket, walked a little like a high-school athlete, launching himself off the balls of his feet, rolling his shoulders, hands in a semi-fist. Only in the most abstract sense was it possible to think of him as small. Though he was often impatient and distracted, I never saw him tired or bored, and only once or twice did I see him at leisure.

The angiography room was at the end of the corridor, and waiting for him there was the other resident who had been at the meeting with Charlie White, José Rivera, a Puerto Rican who, like Benny, had also trained in England.

"What have we got?" Brockman said.

"Mrs. Hennessey, the glioma. And Victor Alfredo, re-member him?"

"That giant aneurysm? Is he back already?"

"He had a seizure last night. They brought him in about three thirty."

"Shit, I didn't expect him back so soon. Let's see him first."

José switched on the screen, then mounted the angio-grams. The aneurysm stood out like a puff of smoke, al-most exploding from the vessel. Brockman whistled.

"That's depressing, isn't it? God knows why it hasn't bled. He won't last six months with that thing in his head. If it doesn't blow, it's gonna push all the way through his temporal lobe. We've got to sell them on an anastomosis."

The reference was to a new technique in which blood vessels are transplanted and the flow of blood redirected.

Smaller aneurysms are usually treated by clipping them off, but Victor's was too big for that. An anastomosis would involve, first, redirecting blood flow from his cranium to the region around the aneurysm, then clipping the vessel from which the aneurysm had grown so as to deprive it of blood. The transplant, if it worked, would replace the blood lost when the vessel was clipped.

"It's obvious he needs an anastomosis," José said, "but I don't know if his family will permit it. Have you met his brother?"

"Yeah, I remember him," Brockman said. "Nothing we can do about him. What can we offer except what we've got on the menu? Let's see the glioma."

José removed Victor's X-rays and searched a pile for Mrs. Hennessey's, but before he found them, Jack Beecham, chief of radiology, poked his head in the door. "Jim, can I speak to you a minute?"

Brockman followed him into the hall. When they returned a few minutes later, there was another man with them, a friend of a friend of Beecham's whose son, age five, was suffering from glioma. He was Duane Kirschner, a jeweler from San Francisco. Surgeons there had called his boy's tumor inoperable, and when he'd asked around for someone who might be willing to go for it, several people had given him Brockman's name. He had flown in last night with the angiograms and the CAT-scans, and now they posted them on the screen.

The tumor was distinct, as frightening as Victor Alfredo's aneurysm. Since it was located in the boy's dominant hemisphere, where removal would produce a neurological deficit too large to contemplate, it was obvious that surgery could not be justified. Brockman must have known this at once, but he spent several minutes with the scans before examining the angiograms, then went back to the scans again. Finally he shook his head. "That's a tough tumor, sir. There's no way in the world we can do it."

Kirschner took a step back and leaned against the wall, then sank into a chair as though all his strength had disappeared. "But you've got to help me," he said.

"Hell, don't you think I'd like to? There's nothing we can do. That tumor . . . look here where it's spread . . . we'd have to take a third of his brain. And even if we did, cells like that . . . they come back too fast. No. God, I'm sorry to say it, but there's really nothing we can do."

Kirschner seemed oblivious to what he'd heard. "Dr. Kravetz, in California, he said if anyone would operate, it would be you. We'll take the chance. We'll expect the worst, I give you my word. You've got to help him. This is my son! Don't you realize . . . don't you know what I'm saying?"

"Of course I know. I understand what you're going through. But we can't go in there and destroy the kid's brain. No way can we do it. The best thing to do is give him radiation. Take these pictures downstairs to Mrs. Calendar and she'll give you an opinion. They can handle his treatment perfectly well in California."

Once again, Kirschner ignored him. He was crying now, leaning with his head in his hands and talking to the floor. "He was such a joyous child. Everybody loved him! We were just starting to play ball together. Then one night he woke up with a headache, and the next morning we couldn't get him out of bed. . . . Kravetz said you'd take the chance."

The situation was impossible. Brockman had a meeting scheduled in fifteen minutes and he still had angiograms to see. He wouldn't get back to radiology until late this evening, after rounds, and before that he had to see the families, like Mrs. Hennessey's and Victor's, who were waiting to see what the X-rays had determined.

Sometimes Brockman got mean, but never with people like this. When he was ready to operate and people balked, when residents messed up, when patients nagged him, he could be merciless, but when the situation was hopeless, like this one, he was riveted, humbled, a little embarrassed, perhaps, by his impotence. Nor did it help that for people in such situations egocentricity was total. For Kirschner, at this moment, there was no one else in the world, no other patient in the hospital, no other demand on the Boss's attention but his son's disease. I think he would have continued like this indefinitely had Beecham not taken him by the arm and led him from the room. "Come on," he said. "Let's go see Mrs. Calendar. Maybe she can help."

Brockman and José watched him go, then gazed in silence for a moment at the empty X-ray screen. They lived with illness, but certain catastrophes affected them as they affect anyone else, and one of those most certain to do so was cancer in a child.

"Some tumor," Brockman said at last. "Jesus, did you see how big that fucker was?" He lit another cigarette, shook his head and then—one of the things he was best at —let it pass. "Let's see the other glioma. I've got a meeting ten minutes ago in administration."

3

A Certain Frame of Mind

Two days after Charlie entered the hospital, he was interviewed by Bryan Margolin, the senior social worker, and invited to attend the Tuesday meetings that he and his assistant, David Getz, conducted in the ward. Ostensibly, these sessions were meant to offer patients a chance to share their experiences and problems, but they also gave Bryan and David an opportunity to forget for a while their principal work (dealing with the social and mechanical problems that illness produces) and explore certain therapeutic fantasies for which, it seemed to me, they had no talent whatsoever.

Social workers don't rank very high in the medical establishment, and their meetings aren't treated with much respect. Conference rooms and large offices were available, but these meetings were held in the ninth-floor Visitors' Lounge opposite the elevators. What with newspaper wagons, oxygen tanks, and breakfast trays rattling up and down the hall, and all sorts of impromptu conferences developing between doctors and nurses while they waited for elevators, distraction was constant. Bryan and David tried to deal with the problem by placing screens between the patients and the elevators, but this was a public lounge and visitors kept peeking, and sometimes they sat down to join the group. The great problem, however, was attendance. Most neurosurgical patients didn't feel like talking, and some couldn't talk at all, but those who could were not what you'd call excited by the idea of this sort of meeting. Bryan and David had to hustle for business every Tuesday, and it seemed to me that most patients who came did so less out of need than of politeness and timidity. Like patients everywhere, they'd do most anything you said if you were wearing a white jacket.

David began the meeting that morning as he always did, with a formula talk that made everyone uptight. "All right, I guess we're all here now. Why don't we begin our meeting? I'll start by explaining our purpose. We've found, Bryan and I, that patients who've been through the neurosurgical experience can help each other by sharing their thoughts and fears. You've all been here different lengths of time. And we know how frightening it is to come on the neurosurgical floor, leaving your jobs and families, facing the trauma of surgery. But we think it helps if you talk about it. Doctors treat you medically, but we want to see how you respond as individuals."

In addition to Charlie, four people were present that morning. Happily for me, one of them was a woman named Rosie Galindez, who had an inexhaustible sense of humor. It was Rosie who took charge of the group that morning and saved it from David. Without Rosie's help, I think no one would have thought of anything to say.

This was the third time Rosie had been admitted to the hospital, once for ostensibly successful surgery on a benign tumor and twice because the wire-mesh plate with which they'd patched her skull had become infected. She was slated for "repair" in three days, but for now her forehead was puffed out like a unicorn's. Repair, though a superficial form of surgery, required reopening the skull, and that meant shaving the head again, anesthesia, another incision, pain, itching, and discomfort later. But I never heard her complain. Like Charlie, she called the whole trip "an adventure" (even, one time, "a very nice experience") and resented anesthesia, she said, because she didn't want to miss "the show."

Such detachment was unusual but not unique on the ward. Those who had it were fortunate, almost blessed, compared with those who didn't. All the patients were caught in their own particular Jobian bind, but the manner in which they took their news was always, to a certain extent, a function of their detachment and sense of humor. Some went to pieces, whined like five-year-olds, and others, their conditions equally hopeless, took it like heroes. Though it was rare to greet news of one's operation with "Dynamite!" the way Charlie White did, the whole range was visibly and very subtly modulated here, humor and stoicism and detachment at one end of the spectrum, whining and self-pity and pure screaming terror at the other. Some patients considered themselves so insignificant and the Boss so celestial that they wouldn't detain him even for urgent questions, while others greeted him on evening rounds like spoiled kids waiting for their father when he came home from work. One complained, "I rang for water today and it was ten minutes before the nurse showed up!" And another, during Passover, "That's the second day in a row they gave me bread instead of matzoh." Some went paranoid, imagined conspiracies among the doctors to leave their tumors inside; others could not comprehend illness except as moral failure. "But I don't understand," said the husband of one patient, when they told him of his wife's tumor. "She was always so good." Not common but not terribly infrequent were people like Rosie, who simply took it and saw it, insisting on their right to clarity, transcending their fear moment by moment through no medium but their humor and attention, their refusal to take themselves too seriously. "It's coming back!" said the Boss one evening to a woman whose leg had been paralyzed for two months after surgery. "Yeah," she said. "So is Christmas."

That sort of humor was easy to take, much-needed comic relief, but sometimes patients' humor drove you up the wall. One fellow I knew had been attacked by a mugger who had caved in his head and also, it seemed, given him a sense of humor. The attack had left him permanently disabled, both brain-damaged and disfigured, with a huge concavity in his forehead. There was little doubt that he would be hospitalized the rest of his life. Although he had always been, according to his wife, rather lazy and indolent, even morose, he was now euphoric and gregarious, entertaining the ward like a stand-up comic. He called the concavity "my ashtray." Like a lot of patients with frontal-lobe damage, he suffered from what they call "duplication," so he was of the opinion that there were two hospitals, one where he was "hanging out" and another, just like it, across the street. He could not understand why he was served six meals every day when all he ate was three. Having discovered, along with his jokes, a large creative impulse, he wanted to paint and write stories (not fiction, though: "I don't like made-up stories because they're fictitious"), and claimed to be working on a novel entitled "Van Gogh: A Wrestler and a Blind Writer." At conference, the staff agreed that he was "confabulating," but as someone noted, "Let us remember that confabulations in the brain-damaged are not appreciably different from those in normal people." And they warned each other not to "reinforce" his confusion. "After all," said one neurologist, "everyone likes a euphoric patient."

Such people could give you strange, uncomfortable sensations, as if the ground beneath you were suddenly insufficient for your weight. Nonpatients, to say the least, brought insecurities to the hospital. It was very important

to distinguish yourself from patients, to keep a good hold
on the illusion that sickness and health are absolutely separate, that what had laid them out was not about to lay you
out as well. Those patients who laughed at their own disease could shake those distinctions and remind you of your
own vulnerability. There was value there if you went with
it; any patient could become a kind of guru if you had the
nerve to listen. If not, the hospital was an obstacle course,
a series of misadventures that sent you reeling with paranoia.

When Rosie led off the meeting that morning in her
particular manner, giving a hilarious account of outsiders
and their ambivalence toward neurosurgical patients (how
they went pale all over while simultaneously trying to
comfort her, how in the end she always had to comfort
them), David tried to laugh but couldn't. Fumbling with his
notebook, his back very straight in his chair, he said, "Isn't
it nice you've kept your sense of humor!"

I thought at first David was putting us on, doing a sort
of social-worker parody, but this was his way of handling
the paranoia. The less secure one's authority (and no authority here was less secure than that of the social
worker), the more threatened one feels by patients who
laugh at themselves, and the greater the need to patronize
them. Humor makes you feel a bit too much aware of your
similarity to the patients. Who can be sure, anyhow, that
one's own brain isn't damaged? That an aneurysm isn't
lurking in your head? If you can get into your work and
your authority, surround yourself with helpless, morbid
patients, you can solidify the wall between yourself and
them. But a patient like Rosie can reveal the wall for what
it is: a delusion, sustained by the power of thought and
social convention but pathetically vulnerable to the whims
of nature and the fragility of the body.

A few weeks later, one patient—a stroke victim—took
me on a trip through my own paranoia. She was new on the

ward and had not seen me before. On the morning we met, the nurse wheeled her in and placed her opposite me in the Visitors' Lounge, and she smiled in such a way that I knew she thought I was a patient (patients do not smile at nonpatients the way they smile at each other). She had not seen me before, so she did not know I could speak, had not seen me walk so as to know I wasn't paralyzed, and since one of the ironies of brain damage is that it often leaves the appearance intact, there was no way for her to see in my face that I was not, like her, a stroke victim. We were alone together for maybe three minutes, but during that time I was brain-damaged in her mind. If in my own I was not, I was at least aware that the decision to call oneself "brain-damaged" or "normal" is itself a function of the brain, requiring (among other things) the memory of such descriptions, the ability to retrieve them, and the motor capacity to articulate them. With that awareness I lost almost completely the "me-them" distinctions I had brought to the hospital. I was not exactly a patient, but I was not exactly not-a-patient either. In fact, it struck me that the region in my brain that called her brain "damaged" might be no less damaged than the region in hers which called it nothing at all.

She continued to smile sweetly, but I felt she was laughing at me. I wanted to stand up and walk around the room just to show her who was boss, to fire questions she could not answer to remind her of her aphasia. But in the midst of the paranoia there was kinship too, compassion that seemed different from what I had called by that name in the past, devoid, I mean, of pity or self-pity, fear for myself or disgust with her (these being, in my experience, the principal components in what is usually called "compassion" for the sick). I didn't really *want* the compassion, but it came upon me anyhow.

It seemed to me that the superiority I had imagined with respect to her was itself a symptom, another kind of brain damage. What's more pathological than attachment to descriptions that contradict reality? In fact, every judgment I made struck me now as a kind of tic, a firing of dysfunctional neurons. The more kinship I felt with her, the more aware I felt of my own brain function, and the more aware of it, the more separate from it. And this was where the effect of her became more than merely threatening. Somehow she had shown me what I had often thought but rarely known, that I was more than my brain, more than the language, thought, and judgment which emanated from my cortex and often obscured everything beyond it. For an instant, indeed, my brain struck me as funny. Brain damage struck me as funny. And then for an instant all the fear I had ever known seemed obsolete. Isn't fear itself, like language and memory, a function of the brain? If you laugh at the brain, view your neurons as capricious, how can any fear remain?

A moment later all of it was gone. David arrived, and then the patient and I were introduced. Nodding, smiling, producing words in proper sequence, I became, as they say, my old self again, and she was whispering what happened to be the only word she had that morning, "Okay, okay, okay." Whatever memory remained in me of the moments before was distant, romantic, and intimidating. If memory is a function of the brain, what is the brain to do with memories of its own diminishment?

Such experiences, conscious or not, transient or not, were common at the hospital, not just for outsiders like me but for people on the staff as well. Patients dissolved your self-defense, and unless you could relinquish it your response to them was paranoid. The crucial thing was how much, on any given day, you could contemplate your own brain, your own absurdity, your own vulnerability and mortality. On uptight days (David, for example, this morning), such thoughts could drive you crazy, but good days could be as rich as any you had ever known. People like

Rosie, on days like that, could release you from your fear of illness and sometimes even your fear of death.

Bryan wasn't too much looser than David. His strategy against paranoia was reinterpretation. He seemed to think it therapeutic for patients if they could hear their own words paraphrased by her. "What you're saying, if I understand you correctly, is that your experience has changed your life. Does anyone else have similar feelings?" He tried to view everything positively, to help patients, against all odds, see things optimistically. "If I may comment, your having surgery was a very brave thing to do. You decided to go for broke. If I were you, sir, I'd be awfully proud of myself." Patients were generally polite with him, but once the group got started, they were so eager to hear from each other and to share what they had to say that they often cut him off or inadvertently put him down.

As it happened, the man sitting opposite him could do that better than anyone on the ward. He was a psychoanalyst named Peter Fleischman, who had an inoperable cancer called astrocytoma (because the cells are shaped like stars), and he was far beyond the point where politeness, or even logic, concerned him. When Bryan began to reinterpret what Rosie had said ("Are you saying that outsiders don't really understand what neurosurgical patients feel?"), he raised his hand and interjected, "All right! What do you feel today and who have you discussed it with?"

"I beg your pardon?" Bryan asked.

Fleischman did not answer. Instead he glared at him as if he were his patient, then went off on a tangent that had no connection with what he had said.

Fleischman's tumor was the most lethal of any that strike the brain. Yesterday the Boss had told his family that there would be no operation, and later today he was going home. In six months he would be dead. This morning, however, he looked, as he often did, radiant and inspired. He was sixty-nine years old, a tall, heavyset fellow with an unkempt white beard he'd grown since falling ill three months before. A well-known psychoanalytic theorist who had published three books and many professional articles, he had been visited, during his time at the hospital, by a continuous procession of colleagues, students, and patients, most of whom left his room in tears. Although he vacillated between lucidity and incoherence, he was always interesting and alert, and sometimes, like a lot of aphasiacs, his linguistic failures were inspired, a combination of Wallace Stevens and Groucho Marx. All his colleagues agreed that his illness had transformed him, but there was considerable disagreement between the romantics, who called him "enlightened," and the rationalists, who called him "sick." "This is a man," said one of the former, "who's struggled all his life to understand, but only in the past two months has he been at peace with himself."

Even among the rationalists, however, there were few who'd argue that his illness had made him a different sort of man. As one of his former patients described him, he had been a man "who believed that the mind could transcend everything, that a problem analyzed correctly would disappear, that nothing lay beyond the powers of thought and understanding." He had pursued psychoanalysis with a fervor that was completely religious, almost fanatical, and he had accepted without qualification its dependence on language and reason. Now he was unable to trust either. All that he believed in had suddenly betrayed him. How had it affected him? "For the first time," said one of his colleagues, "he seems vulnerable and accessible. He was charismatic before, almost intimidating. His assumption always seemed to be that he was beyond everyday phenomena. Now he's stripped, frightened, absolutely real. He talks to you about himself, laughs like a child, cries when he's scared. It's as if the tumor has freed him to become a member of the human community."

Fleischman himself, though sometimes he was frightened ("What will they do with me?"), sided mostly with the romantics. Like Charlie White's, his tumor was something of an ego trip. On the slightest pretext, he would relate the most intimate stories from his past as if he were a patient in analysis. Mostly, as I say, he considered himself transformed and liberated and, in the Buddhist sense, completely enlightened.

"What you see before you," he told me once, "is the same thing that happened with that fellow—what was his name?—in fifth-century India. This sort of thing only happens every five or ten thousand years. Everyone who comes to see me is more serene and tranquil, more fulfilled. It's nothing to do with me, mind you. Something else is working in me, just as it worked with Buddha—yes, that's the name! How long have you been here, for example? See? You don't know. Time disappears in my presence!"

At Fleischman's funeral, six months later, one of his colleagues, a Japanese psychoanalyst, gave a eulogy which accepted the romantic interpretation of his condition. "I have spent time in my native country with Zen masters and I can say to you without qualification that in his last months Dr. Fleischman attained the ultimate state of enlightenment which in Zen is called satori."

Whether he was enlightened or sick, there was no question that Fleischman, unlike a lot of patients on the ward, was detached in relation to his disease, almost awesome in his equanimity. "I have my perception of what is happening," he said later that day, before he went home. "It's different from the doctors', but that's all right. It's not a question of good or bad. If they need to know more about it from the outside, let them go ahead with their tests. What I have to do is follow it deeper and deeper inside, to be quiet and get into it until it resolves itself in another way. The time is coming when I won't speak at all. I will begin to close down more and more, and that will be the end. I accept and I hope. I wish I could say to you what my feeling about dying is, but I can only say what it is not: not good or bad, not welcome or unwelcome. It is. I am it. I am in a condition of secondlessness."

I asked him if he could explain what he meant by "secondlessness," and he looked at the ceiling, shaking his head.

"Secondlessness?" he said. "Oh, no. I couldn't do that."

All these statements were made during moments when he was relatively lucid. Brain tumors, especially astrocytomas, swell and exert pressure on healthy cells surrounding them, and since his tumor was in his left temporal lobe, both his language and memory were affected—erratically and unpredictably. Often he wouldn't remember me when I came to visit, and sometimes he'd become incoherent, drifting off into distracted whispers, or simply go round the bend.

When David turned to Fleischman that morning and asked how he was feeling, he clenched his fist and gritted his teeth and made a sound like a growling dog. "Sometimes . . . mad as hell . . . grr! But sometimes"—he broke into a grin—"light as a feather! Happy as a bird!"

"Do you think you could explain that a little more?" Bryan asked.

"Well, that depends on how you look at it. You take England. Two thousand, three thousand years, and now . . . no water! Israel . . . Syria . . . same problem. Who can say? Who can say?"

"England?" Rosie cried. "What's England got to do with it?"

Fleischman didn't answer. Looking upward, his face took on its familiar radiance, and he seemed to drift off into the stratosphere.

He didn't say much more that morning, but the gaps he left were more than adequately filled by the man sitting next to me, a former schoolteacher named Raymond Dreyer whose surgery, two weeks before, had left him with a form of aphasia that turns language into endless circumlocution. No one was going to suggest that Mr. Dreyer was "enlightened." From any point of view he was zonked out, shell-shocked, and he'd never get better. Like Fleischman's, his tumor was in his left temporal lobe. It was a bit more advanced, also an astrocytoma, but in his case they'd tried for a partial removal in order to relieve some of his more bizarre symptoms. He was a little better than before surgery, but he'd never be lucid or detached or high on his illness, and his language would always be a mix of descending circles, less Groucho Marx than Richard Nixon at his most outrageous, a remarkable parody, it seemed to me, of the Oval Office tapes.

"Excuse me for interrupting," Dreyer said, when Fleischman drifted off, "but I don't mean to be argumentative. I requested the doctor examine me. I'm not saying this in vain, or knocking the doctors, you understand? Every time they said high blood pressure, low blood sugar, now that really frightened me, you understand? I don't mean to criticize. It frightened me emotionally, physically, morally. The minute you're involved with the head, you're involved with mystery. That's how I understand it, if you'll excuse the interruption. Where it comes to a tumor, a cancer, a brain, it's a lack of experience. I don't mean to knock anyone, you understand, but—"

Rosie interrupted him. "Wait a minute, why can't you complain?"

"Complain? Who's complaining?" Dreyer said.

"Listen . . . what's your name anyhow?"

Having lost his name six weeks before, Dreyer turned to Bryan for help.

"His name is Mr. Dreyer," he said. "Raymond Dreyer."

"Well, listen here, Raymond, if you can't complain now, you never can. If I were you I'd complain at the top of my voice! Let 'em hear it! You've got more to complain about than anyone I ever met!"

There was laughter at this, great relief, but none from Bryan or Dreyer. Bryan seemed more and more uptight, as though the laughter foretold the group's disintegration. Now he dipped into his psychiatric bag and came up with another parody of a social worker. "Mr. Dreyer," he said, to a man who'd recently lost nearly 15 percent of his brain, "do you feel insecure?"

"Hell yes, he's insecure!" Rosie cried. "Why shouldn't he be?"

Dreyer slumped in his chair as if defeated, but there was a hint of a smile at the corner of his mouth. He was a small, wiry man who looked as if he once might have been an athlete, his skin slightly blue like that of many patients on the ward. At each temple he bore the rust-colored cross-marks which the radiation therapist had applied to guide his machine and repeat its angles from day to day so that the radiation (which everyone knew to be useless in Dreyer's case) would hit his tumor instead of the healthy cells around it. He wore the beige watch cap they gave to everyone when they shaved their heads before surgery, but his was slightly askew, tipped jauntily toward his forehead, so you could see the long zipper of a scar curving upward from the base of his skull. In the bright light of the Visitors' Lounge he looked less like a human being than an imitation of one, a figure in a wax museum, a heavy-handed sculpture by an artist out to portray the absurdity of existence.

David leaped into the silence to defend the group against Dreyer, who would have talked all day if no one had stopped him. There were two patients we had yet to hear, both of them a bit easier on the eye and mind than Dreyer and Fleischman, and he turned to them now as if for relief.

Some relief. One was Charlie, his head not yet shaved, his eyes wide with terror at the psychodrama that Fleischman and Dreyer had staged for him, and the other was his roommate, George Tinker, who was five days postop, as the vernacular goes, after surgery on a meningioma that had been similar in some respects to Charlie's.

David tried to draw Charlie into the conversation, but he hadn't much to say. Though paler since the night we'd met, he was well on his way toward the self-importance which, after his surgery, would become extreme, the sense of his tumor as a "mission" and a "test." It was an intricate, slightly hysterical, big-game philosophy that would help him not a little to deal with his illness. Every once in a while, as now, he cringed beneath a thought as if someone's fingernails had scratched a blackboard in his mind, but quicker than any other patient I had met, he shook it off and found another slogan to help him on his way. Mostly, these consisted of the sort of platitudes one ought to keep to oneself, but since there were usually people around his bed and he was, for the time being, the center of attention, he could not restrain himself. "This is a great challenge," he'd say. "I'm gonna stand tall, watch and see, I'm gonna come through this with flying colors."

Like a lot of patients with neurological disease, Charlie was convinced he had a book in him. He wrote constantly in a notebook he kept beside his bed, and he'd bought himself a tape recorder so that, with Roberta's help, he could tape what he said after surgery, when he came up from anesthesia. "Years from now," he explained, "I'll be able to listen to it. What a pisser! It'll be like hearing myself being born!" When he weakened, he was terrified, obsessed with every change in his condition, desperate to explain why this had happened. "Was it my diet, do you think? I always ate a lot of junk food." But a moment later he would turn it around again, flash a grin a bit too broad, and say he was "thankful" for his illness. Once, only half in jest, he expressed gratitude because it had given him, a suburban boy, a chance to spend a night in the big city. When someone asked, the night before his surgery, if he was afraid, he gave what seemed to me an apt description of the mental gymnastics in which he was engaged. "The way I look at it, it's only a matter of getting my head in a certain frame of mind."

Mostly, I liked being with him, but he was hard to take when he got pretentious and romantic about his tumor. Impressed as I was by his courage and his lack of self-pity, I had seen enough neurosurgery to know what he was eulogizing, and as a writer I recoiled at his language as I had expected to recoil in the operating room. We like to think disease brings out the eloquence, the poetry, in people, but if clichés and platitudes lurk in the mind, serious illness will draw them out as quickly as alcohol or marijuana. As an English teacher, Charlie was not insensitive to language, but he was so desperate to understand and articulate what had happened to him that he had left his critical judgment at the door of the hospital. Worse yet, no one could tell him, as they would outside, to slow down a bit, leave a thing or two unsaid. That's just one of the games that healthy people play with the sick, just one of the reasons why sick people, as Rosie remarked, find it so difficult to trust the well. "Once they know you're sick," she said, "no one tells you the truth about yourself, not even the doctors."

Charlie's roommate, George Tinker, had expressed similar resentment. In fact, so often did he return to the subject that it seemed primary among all the pains his illness had produced. Considering that George's recent operation had been his third encounter with neurosurgery in the past twelve years, that he had been a patient in three of the greatest neurosurgical hospitals (one of them in Canada) and that his surgeons had been three of the best who had ever lived, and, finally, that his illness had taken him through almost every dysfunction that can afflict the central nervous system, his opinions had to be a sort of gospel. And principal among the agonies he had suffered was the paranoia his illness had produced. "Except for my wife, there was no one I trusted completely. Everyone else seemed to be watching me for signs, telling me what they thought I wanted to hear, feeling sorry for me or frightened of me, expecting me to fail or hoping I would. I thought it was bad when I went to the hospital, but it was when I went back to work that my troubles really began."

When David realized that Charlie wouldn't help him much to keep the meeting lively, he turned his attention to George. Nowhere on the ward could he have found a better ally. One question was all it took to set him off on a sort of travelogue through neurosurgery, the differences between this surgeon and that, the Boss and his Canadian counterparts, the advances in treatment during the years since his first illness. And when he finished, he went back to the beginning and took us step by step through the illness which, for the last fifteen years, had tyrannized his life.

George was forty-four years old, stocky and muscular, with sad brown eyes and a quizzical expression that any stranger would know was earned. His first seizure had come when he was thirty-one. Until that moment he had been the sort of fellow who thought he had never been sick a day in his life, though he'd been accident-prone since infancy. A fine athlete who had played the National Junior Tennis Championships at Forest Hills and quarterback at Dartmouth, he was finally banned from all sports at college after his nose had been broken seven times and he had suffered three brain concussions. No one would ever know whether those concussions had played a part in the tumors which eventually formed in his brain. One of the surgeons who treated him for his first tumor suggested it had been present at birth, but such is the nature of tumor research that there was no more evidence for that than for the concussions or, for that matter, the psychological trauma which had dominated his life during the two years preceding his seizures.

Though far from conclusive, some recent research has drawn connections between psychological stress and traumatic illness like Hodgkin's disease or stroke or brain tumor. It seems that many victims of such disease have suffered extreme disorientations—the loss of a loved one, for instance, or a catastrophic setback in career—during the two or three years preceding the onset of their symptoms. Nothing conclusive, as I say, but George Tinker, like a number of patients I met, made those theories look awfully good. At twenty-nine, he had been edging into the American Dream, moving toward the vice-presidency of a large corporation, his wife pregnant with their second child, living in a fashionable suburb, bowling two nights a week, playing tennis, coaching a Little League baseball team. Two years later he had been through what he called "a lifetime of problems": the child was born brain-damaged, developed meningitis, and died six months later; his father had a stroke on the same day his father-in-law learned that he was dying of cancer; he bought a house he couldn't pay for in a desperate attempt to help him and his wife forget their dead child; his father-in-law died; his father, paralyzed by the stroke, developed a pathological dependency which made it impossible for him to sleep at night unless George visited him.

In the summer of 1963, a month after his third child's birth, George felt a weakness in his leg while mowing the lawn. Of course he ignored it. ("Why?" Rosie asked, and George shrugged. "Why not? Jesus, at that point in my life, I considered myself immortal.") The denial, common among neurological patients (not to mention the rest of us), would continue throughout his illness.

A few weeks later, he noticed an inexplicable loss of

hearing, increasing weakness in his leg, and once, in September, his leg gave way completely. He mentioned these symptoms to no one. Only when his leg began to misbehave absurdly, straighten and kick and go into spasms, often in front of other people, did he finally see a doctor, but the internist he chose found nothing. Three weeks later, his right leg stiffened on the accelerator of his car and caused it to race ahead until he thought to remove it with his left foot. During those three weeks, his bowling average had dropped by 100 points and his tennis game had gone to pieces. Like many patients on this ward, George often measured the ravages of his disease by its effect on his athletic skills.

Returning one afternoon from a business trip, he went out to dinner, went bowling, came home exhausted, and, as his head touched the pillow, had his first convulsion, what doctors call a grand mal seizure. "Blotto" was what George called it. "My legs went rigid and my arms flailed and my head stretched backward on the pillow." His wife had the presence of mind to protect him from biting his tongue, but unfortunately she did it with her thumb. By the time his seizure had subsided and the ambulance was on its way, there were gashes on the top and bottom of her thumb and her blood was all over the bed.

The first doctor they called was the internist who had examined George three weeks before. He told him to take two aspirin and go to bed. A bit dubious about such advice, they called the family pediatrician and got the name of a neurologist, Dr. John Symondson, who told them to get to the hospital at once. At the hospital, George had another seizure, this one striking, as the other had, when he placed his head on the pillow. When he woke the next morning, Dr. Symondson was standing over his bed. It is some measure of the progress in neurology—since George's disease would not be particularly difficult to diagnose these days —that the first thing Symondson did was confess his ignorance to him. "There's ninety-nine percent about neurology that I don't know, but if the one percent I do know applies to your problem, I would say I have about a fifty percent chance of finding out what's wrong."

Seizures are generally associated with epilepsy, but they can be caused by any scar or dysfunction in the brain. There is not much agreement among researchers as to their exact etiology. They are caused by an abnormal firing of neurons, a chemical or electrical disorder which, if strong enough, can affect adjacent cells and, in the case of grand mal seizures, proliferate until large portions of the brain are involved.

Like most seizure victims, George could catalog his attacks with relentless precision, and no wonder: since that first convulsion, his life had been dominated by seizures and the memory of seizures and, worst of all, the anticipation of seizures. "It got so I never knew, when I put my foot down, where it would end up." Thus, there was the time when he went to visit his mother in the hospital and, while trying to convince her to eat her dinner, flipped upside down in a grand mal seizure that left, he swears, his footprint on the ceiling. Coming to, on the floor, he heard himself: "You've got to eat!" and his mother, from her bed: "Where are you?" Or the afternoon in Newark when a seizure in a parking lot left him, mute and paralyzed and with a broken heel, in the path of a truck backing up that stopped not twelve inches from his face. Or the time he was alone in a hotel room in Miami, or the many times in automobiles, or the time he fell twenty steps at Madison Square Garden, or the time he was swimming and was carried helpless by the surf a quarter mile up the beach.

As Dostoevski made us realize, seizures are an ultimate metaphor for ontological insecurity, one way quicker than any other that our bodies can remind us of our helplessness before Nature. Sometimes George claimed he could control a seizure with "thought," and sometimes he called his own claim ridiculous. He often observed the seizure as if from afar, as if in slow motion, and had very clear thoughts while falling, admonishing himself, for example, to protect his head, or arranging already for help. "If I tried to control it physically, I made it worse, but sometimes, if I told myself, Don't let it go any further, it seemed to work."

As with most epileptics, his seizures were often preceded by an aura, a physical sensation either vivid or vague, bright lights, a foul smell, dizziness, sometimes a burning on his back, very often a brief loss of hearing, even more often a tap on the back of his thigh. Sometimes his limbs went out in all directions, sometimes his body went rigid and he slid slowly to the floor. Frequently he went unconscious, numb on one side, and there was a long period when he ground his teeth so violently that he damaged his jaw.

There were peaceful seizures and violent seizures, terrifying seizures and seizures that brought clarity and radiance. They were as much a part of George's life as his heartbeat, essential factors in every plan he made, handicaps on any job he took, cruel threats in the back of his mind, dues to pay—since they were amazingly responsive to psychological stress—when he grew impatient or anxious or angry at himself or paranoid or lonely or insecure with his friends. Drugs could control them, up to a point (Symondson told him that first day that he'd be on pills the rest of his life), but there were dues to pay for them as well. Dilantin—a modern miracle as far as seizure control is concerned—destroys the gums, and phenobarbital plays all sorts of games with one's consciousness, and one never knows what either of them will do to one's energy levels. In any event, the dosage was always a problem. Both he and the doctors tried to shave it as close as they could without leaving room for seizures, but seizures were the only way to know they'd gone too far, and that was costly diagnosis indeed. The worst thing about seizures is that they cause brain damage themselves, thus increasing the likelihood of seizures in the future.

Bryan questioned George about his past, but his answers were elusive. Once he said that after his first operation, which was performed three weeks after his initial convulsion, he had had no seizures at all for seven years, but a moment later he said he had had one nine months later. The former memory was used to support a general, certainly justified feeling that his employers had treated him unfairly after his first operation, the hurt he felt, even these many years later, that after surviving the surgery he had come upon the worst effects of his disease when it was supposedly cured. When he returned to work too soon, half bald still and too proud to wear a wig, his colleagues gave him a party, but toward the end of it his boss took him aside and said, "Go sit in the corner a couple of years, okay? Then we'll reevaluate you." After that, though he worked desperately to compensate and prove himself, he was turned down for promotions he ought to have received. Worse, he developed a sense that people were watching him, shaking their heads when he turned his back. An old habit of leaning his head on one hand while writing became a liability. "I wouldn't do that," his boss said. "It looks like you're holding it because it's sore." He denied then, as he denied at our morning meeting, that he was ill or incapacitated in any way—"They said I fell down a lot, but I think they were making it up"—but when Bryan pressed him he acknowledged unexplained bruises on his arms and shoulders, a bump now and then on the head. "Who knows?" he said. "Maybe I did fall."

Brockman was by no means insensitive to this dimension of his work, the social and psychological ramifications of brain surgery, the specter it raises in the minds of others. It was always taken into account when determining whether patients were ready to go home, or return to work, or for that matter whether their life situation could tolerate surgery at all. Once, a well-known politician was admitted with a subdural hematoma, a relatively minor (at least in the spectrum of neurosurgical horrors) blood clot on the surface of the brain. Within ten days of the operation, he was doing well enough to go home, but the Boss advised him to stay away from the office. "Your enemies will be watching you for signs of brain damage. If I were you I'd take a vacation until my hair grew back."

How George's colleagues saw him was a matter of argument, but there was no argument about the bitterness he felt or the alienation it produced. Four years after surgery, he was offered an annual disability pension of $10,000 if he would retire, but he turned it down. A year later he quit in anger, with no pension, set up his own (advertising) business, and miraculously made a go of it for several years, until he was finally forced to admit that he'd become a full-fledged epileptic.

The admission did not come easily. Nine years after his first operation, he still thought of himself as a man in reasonably good health. True, he was having seizures almost all the time, but his capacity for denial remained vigorous, and he had blind faith in Symondson, a doctor of the old school who, like a lot of neurologists, distrusted surgery and still believed that George could be controlled with drugs.

Around that time, however, George finally complied with his wife's wishes that he see a psychiatrist. More clearly and objectively than George, she had seen what was happening to him, the paranoia and the uncertainty, the guilt he felt about his inadequacies at work, the effect of his illness on their children (his daughter had nightmares for years about a seizure George had when no one but he and she were home).

When the psychiatrist—a woman in her late forties named Sarah Collins—entered the picture, George found himself in a triangle that was universal in American medicine. With neurosurgery perched on the distant horizon like a panacea, a concrete one-step solution which at times could seem almost romantic, neurology and psychiatry submitted their own adamant interpretations of his predicament. The more Symondson espoused Dilantin and phenobarbital, the more Collins sought to get him off drugs entirely. It was her opinion that, in addition to keeping him constantly fatigued, they were masking his real symptoms and serving as a dangerous psychological crutch, a means of "avoiding responsibility."

There were meetings at the hospital where one could see this triangle displayed with almost comic predictability. At the same hour every Tuesday afternoon, psychiatrists, neurologists, and neurosurgeons gathered to present selected patients to one another (to determine, among other things, whether a patient was acting crazy because he had something wrong with his brain or acting as if he had something wrong with his brain because he was crazy), and it always seemed to me that anyone with the slightest knowledge of the medical profession would have known the surgeons from the neurologists and the psychiatrists from both. For me it became a sort of game to see if I could identify new people—young residents, for instance, or visitors not on the regular staff—and I was almost never wrong. You could identify the neurosurgeons because they shared among other things an ability to project themselves that the others seemed to lack. In general, if not unanimously, they were self-confident, men of good carriage and posture who presented their cases as fine athletes present themselves when they come out on the court or the playing field. They were cocky and attractive in their arrogance, and they seemed to like the sound of their own voices, to relish their problems because they believed in their solutions. Very rarely were they self-conscious. If they were concerned about your opinion of them, they did not reveal it to you and more than likely did not reveal it to themselves. As Benny explained, "We almost have to be egomaniacs. Our margins of error are so small and the pressure so great that we'll collapse if we don't have absolute confidence in ourselves. That's why our preparations are so meticulous. We don't leave any room for doubt. If general surgeons prepared as we do, their results would be fantastic." It was the pressure of working within the limited space of the skull, on tissue that is volatile and often indispensable, that made neurosurgeons, on the one hand, so hyperactive and fastidious, on the other, so aggressive. If they didn't lack uncertainty, they had grown so used to it that they were almost indifferent to its effects.

It was easy to see why television thrives on stories about neurosurgeons, or surgeons in general, and why, in contrast, a TV show about a psychiatrist or a neurologist would seem as undramatic as a textbook. Moving along this spectrum, one accumulated self-consciousness and doubt like a boot trudging through mud, and with these burdens came their usual effects on posture and voice, the melancholy, the tortured, hyperconceptual language. Consider the difference between describing a brain tumor and describing a "schizoid tendency," and you'll see why the surgeons sounded so lucid and articulate and the psychiatrists so vague, irresolute, and convoluted. If neurosurgeons were athletes, neurologists would be sportswriters, and psychiatrists that particular sort of arcane philosopher who writes about "sport."

How could it be otherwise? Neurosurgeons deal with patients who are either treated or sent home, neurologists deal mostly with degenerative disease—stroke, for example, or parkinsonism, or senile dementia—which is usually incurable, and psychiatrists treat diseases that are abstract, capricious, intangible, and sometimes, alas, invisible, patients who on any given day can seem absolutely well. If neurosurgeons occupy the real world, psychiatrists occupy a gray area between the real and the illusory, a world in which one can never be completely sure whether a patient is malingering or "really sick," and neurologists —God help them—work somewhere in yet another world between them; parkinsonism, after all, can drive a person crazy, and acute schizophrenics can sometimes behave as if they have parkinsonism.

The triangle is not unrelated to the ubiquitous mind-brain conundrum. Neurosurgeons try their best to ignore behavior (though their work has a nasty way of bringing them full circle), treat the brain as an object, pretend that their work has nothing to do with the mind, but psychiatrists and neurologists are denied this crafty solution: opening the head is not their business. Thus, they are forced to deal with all that lies beyond the concrete particulars of the organism, and that means acknowledging the mind. Their medium is consciousness—language and memory and emotion—and this sends them spinning, no matter how much they discipline their tests and procedures, on the arc between the material and the immaterial. To put it simply, neurosurgeons work in space and psychiatrists in time, and neurologists work in a crazy amalgam of the two, a space-time continuum, if you like. If the principal role of surgeons consists of removing dilemmas from time, locating them entirely in space, the neurologists would seem to be working on a bridge between space and time, with the psychiatrists denied the hope or dream of space at all.

Not surprisingly, the relationship between the three is often politicized. There are surgeons, like Brockman, who are known to favor aggressive treatment of certain kinds of illness (glioma, for example), and neurologists who favor conservatism, sometimes acquiescence—one famous neurologist was known for this pronouncement: "The man's lived long enough, turn him over to the neurosurgeons!"—even with easily manageable conditions like meningioma. Most large medical centers are dominated by either one or the other, and just as a conservative chief of neurology would never permit someone like the Boss to invade his territory, Brockman had done everything he could to assure himself a sympathetic chief of neurology.

In American hospitals the last word, more often than not, belongs to the neurosurgeons. ("They beat on my boys," complained one of the neurologists at Osler Memorial. "I have trouble getting my residents to go over to check on patients they've sent to surgery themselves.") When all other things are equal, the scales are tipped in their favor by the fact that they are trained in neurology and are not ignorant in psychiatry, but neither neurologists nor psychiatrists are trained in neurosurgery. As one of the surgeons put it, playing the ultimate trump card, "If we go down to neurology, we can do everything they do. What can they do if they come up here? Can we let them operate?"

Curiously, this political configuration seems to be an American phenomenon. Residents who have studied in England report the situation there reversed. Neurosurgery is a unit in the neurology ward, and neurologists, though they refer patients to surgery, handle preoperative and postoperative care. "Over there," Benny said, "the surgeon is more or less a handyman."

Some of this is historical. Harvey Cushing, generally recognized as the father of neurosurgery, was American, and most present-day neurosurgeons—American or English—descend from him. In contrast, neurology—marked by great British scientists like Hughlings Jackson and Charles Sherrington—has been an English tradition since its birth as an independent discipline in the nineteenth century. No one can say how much the differences derive from the respective cultures, but the fact remains—as any resident familiar with both situations would confirm—that the "activist, interventionist" discipline of neurosurgery is considered an American specialty, and noninterventionist neurology is distinctly British. "In England," said Benny, "the whole sense in neurology is that you're working on the supreme organ, that you're therefore the supreme physician. They pride themselves on their knowledge of art and literature, their classical education. Over here ... well, there's a tendency toward materialism that makes us all a bit one-sided."

Cultural or historical, medically justifiable or psychologically inevitable, the drama was reenacted at these conferences every Tuesday afternoon. From my point of view, I had to admit that, as a writer, dragging my brain-mind obsessions like luggage when I came to the hospital, I had more in common with the psychiatrists and neurologists than the surgeons. But where my thoughts went, my heart did not follow. It was the surgeons I envied, the surgeons I preferred to sit with when I went to lunch in the cafeteria, the surgeons I wanted to write about. Not for nothing had I been a sports fan all my life. And what fan would sit down with sportswriters and philosophers when the ballplayers themselves were available?

George Tinker had wandered about in this triangle until events made his confusion irrelevant. Although he had little respect for his psychiatrist and unlimited faith in his neurologist, it was Dr. Collins in the end, not Dr. Symondson, who made him (albeit unintentionally) face the truth about himself. Her principal ally was his hatred of medication. After several months of psychotherapy, she convinced him to experiment a little with his Dilantin and phenobarbital. The results were disastrous. Almost at once his seizures increased, and when he resumed his original doses, they did not respond. In fact, he developed a new seizure: up to twenty times a day his mouth would open wide and remain frozen as if in a yawn for up to thirty seconds. Of all his symptoms, he said (looking for some reason at Peter Fleischman, staring at him as if there were no one else in the room), he found these the most embarrassing and frightening and—finally—the most irrefutable. "At last it began to dawn on me that this was not the way to live."

The CAT-scan had not yet been invented, but other tests revealed no tumor. This meant that—as an epileptic—only two forms of treatment were available to him. One was drugs, which Symondson continued to recommend, and the other was seizure surgery, a radical approach which had been pioneered by Wilder Penfield at Montreal's Neurological Institute in the 1930s. If Symondson was antipathetic to neurosurgery in general, he was horrified at the thought of seizure surgery. "They make you look like an experiment," he said. "You'll come out of there a vegetable."

For a while, George heeded his advice (it is hard to appreciate, if you're healthy, the dependency the chronically ill develop on their physician), but one day, during a routine examination, Symondson admitted that he'd never had George "under control." That confession, George said, changed his life. He had two black eyes at the time from falls, a gash on his chin, and he never began a sentence any more without fear that his mouth would freeze before he was done, but until that moment his belief in Symondson had sustained him in his bizarre capacity for optimism. Two weeks later, he and his wife and her mother left for Montreal. Explaining the shift, George put the whole matter in the surreal perspective of his life, describing the collapse of a point of view in language that only a man of his condition and history would have chosen: "When Symondson admitted he couldn't control me, his argument fell out of bed."

The first thing the doctors in Canada did was take him off drugs entirely (they were aghast at the size of his daily dose), and this provoked another sort of crisis—one which, however, had been brewing for years. No neurological disease is without its psychological component, and George's psychology focused principally in a generalized suspicion, in others and sometimes in himself, that none of his seizures were "real." "I'd suspected it all along," he told us that morning, "but in Montreal it came to a head. Way back, when I'd get muscle spasms or lose coordination, I'd tell my wife, 'There's no way to believe this is real.' Me, I'd always felt there was something down underneath, but sometimes it was easier, and maybe less frightening, to think there wasn't. Like maybe I was crazy, you know what I mean?"

In Montreal, the suspicions were seemingly confirmed. For eleven days, without help from Dilantin, there were no seizures at all. Even his electroencephalograph—a dependable tool for tracking epileptic activity—was normal. And slowly, heads began to turn in his direction, slightly quizzical, a touch sad, more than a little angry. "It could be," said one of the doctors, "that you're one out of fifty where we can't track the source, but then again . . ."

As seizure-free time continued, more and more sentences were left unfinished like that. They planned to give him three weeks, then send him home if he'd had no seizures. On the eleventh day, at breakfast, his mother-in-law offered the last of the unfinished sentences: "I don't know, George, I've always thought this was real, but . . ."

Half an hour later, he slid off his chair and convulsed with the biggest seizure of his life. "After that," he said, "I guess she was a believer."

The next EEG showed seizure activity in his left frontal lobe (the area where his first tumor had grown), a region in the brain which, for all its behavioral responsibilities, is not off limits for surgical approach. They gave him two days to make up his mind, but like a lot of patients he didn't need two minutes. He would not have been in Montreal had he not wanted surgery.

"Didn't you even hesitate?" asked Bryan, who knew

something about the risks of seizure surgery. "Weren't you worried about the danger at all?"

"Worried?" George laughed. "The only danger was survival, and I didn't have survival on my mind. What I wanted was a normal life."

Unlike other types of neurosurgery, the Montreal procedure required that patients remain awake so as to answer questions while surgeons probed their brains with electrodes and thus mapped out their neurological functions. As the electrode was moved around the brain and various centers identified, they were labeled with paper tags which the surgeons called "tickets." At the end of the operation the exposed brain looked not a little like a half-completed number painting. The purpose of all this was to excise the dysfunctional cells (providing that, like a large part of the brain, they were not essential) which were causing the epileptic discharge. Ideally, one area, when probed, would trigger a seizure, and once that tiny group of cells had been removed, the epilepsy would be cured.

What was fascinating about the work in Montreal was the information it had produced on brain localization. Never before had it been possible to observe living human brains directly, but now, for the first time, much was tested that had long been theory. Imagine the excitement in the operating room when stimulation in one region of the brain produced a tingling in the thumb or partial blindness or temporary paralysis, all of which disappeared as soon as the electrode was removed. But imagine, too, the mystery one encountered as the electrode moved toward the speech centers and its effects became, as Wilder Penfield put it, "more psychical." One patient was shown a picture of a butterfly while the electrode was applied to his speech cortex. For some time he remained silent, snapping his fingers several times in frustration. When the electrode was withdrawn he cried, "Now I can talk! Butterfly! I couldn't get the word 'butterfly' so I tried to get the word 'moth.' "

When the surgeon's electrode was placed on the interpretive cortex, however, its principal effect was the activation of memories, specific, vivid, and seemingly autonomous. Penfield called it a "doubling of awareness . . . two streams of consciousness flowing, the one driven by input from the environment, the other by the electrode." Of all the information derived from seizure surgery, this has been the most dramatic. Although recent advances in memory research make it seem rather limited, these concrete effects on psychical events fueled the fires on all sides of the brain-mind controversy. Penfield himself found in his data a confirmation of a dualistic position on the brain-mind problem, a conclusion that the brain and mind are separate, that "although the content of consciousness depends in large measure on neuronal activity, awareness itself does not." His principal example was a young South African patient who expressed astonishment on the operating table when he realized that he was laughing with his cousins on a farm in South Africa while he was conscious of being in an operating room in Montreal. "The mind of the patient," wrote Penfield, "was as independent of the [electrode] as was the mind of the surgeon."

Such conclusions, of course, are debatable. Even Penfield admitted that there are many areas of the brain which the electrode cannot explore. The jury remained out after the Montreal discoveries, as it may well remain out forever. And people like George Tinker, when they were rolled in and opened up for the eight-hour spectacular that was the featured attraction in Montreal, couldn't care less.

All that time George was curled like a fetus on his right side, feet tucked, both hands at his chest. There was a sheet between him and the surgeons, but the anesthetist sat next to him and acted as an intermediary. He felt no pain and no particular anxiety when he heard "bones crunching." Occasionally he heard his surgeon's voice just outside the sheet, inches from his ear. "Tell me what you feel now." And then his leg would jump an inch or two, or he would feel a tingling in his arm. Behind the surgeon, another voice, this one on a loudspeaker: "Ask him about 'Right-Four.' " And his right eyelid flickered as if in spasm. Seven hours they continued like this, and then another voice said, "All right, let's close you up," and that was it. He was conscious as they rolled him out, free of pain, and feeling nothing in particular as far as he remembered. In the recovery room a resident asked if he could list the days of the week, and he didn't know where to begin.

There were two good days, and then the seizures came. Early in the afternoon of the third day he had the first, and then, almost at once, another, and then another. Eight full days of seizures ensued. ("When I came to I'd think, Gotta get through this, everything's gonna end up happy. Then I'd have another one.") For eight days they kept his bed in the hall where the nurses could watch him and be ready to jam the tongue depressor in his mouth, and for eight days there were no answers when the doctors quizzed him. Then it was over, as suddenly as it had begun, and everything was back. No seizures, no problems with the doctors' questions; he ate, walked the halls, and two days later they sent him to console another patient, a doctor who was scheduled for the following morning ("I couldn't do it. The guy was hysterical"). No one, as he recalled, bothered to tell him during those eight days that his problems were due to swelling of his brain.*

It was all forgotten when George went home, and once again the measure was athletics. Within three weeks his bowling average, which had dropped to 97 before surgery, climbed to 147, and once, one joyous night, he went over

---

* At that time, steroids (one of the great advances of recent years) were not available to keep edema under control.

200. For the first time in two years he beat his son at tennis. Socializing, an agony since the beginning of his illness, became at least tolerable now, and his vision, off badly the last three years, improved remarkably.

But for all the bliss he knew, the premonitions never ceased. ("All that time," he said, "I never believed it could last.") Two years after the Montreal surgery, his coordination began to disintegrate again, and late that fall, as he stood up to leave a business meeting in Chicago, he collapsed with his first seizure in almost three years. When he got home he had a CAT-scan (the technology was now perfected), and the neurologist, a resident at the hospital, said, "Hey, man, you got problems." Like Charlie White's, the tumor this time was in the rear of his brain, just on the edge of the motor strip.

That's why George was sitting in a wheelchair with us, at our meeting in the Visitors' Lounge. "Don't worry about your arms or your speech," the Boss had told him when he looked at his X rays, "but I can't promise anything about your legs." His right leg was useless to him now, and despite intensive physiotherapy over the next six months, it would never again be dependable. Tennis and bowling were joys of the past, but they were hardly uppermost in his mind. Three days ago, the Boss had told him that this tumor had been malignant (with meningiomas this term doesn't indicate a tendency to spread, as other malignant tumors do, but a predilection for rapid recurrence and invasiveness), and so he, too, like Raymond Dreyer, had radiation crossmarks at his temples.

It was twelve fifteen by now. The meeting had lasted thirty minutes longer than scheduled, and the midday parade was moving through the ward. Brockman and Kellogg, fifteen minutes apart, had come up from surgery to meet with families who had been waiting in the Visitors' Lounge, and a patient with an aneurysm had been taken downstairs, where Harvey would operate on him later this afternoon. Lunch had arrived on tall aluminum carts that looked like erector sets: tuna fish salad, vegetable soup, rice pudding for dessert.

Concluding his tale, George leaned back in his wheelchair and studied the rest of us, waiting for questions. None came. Peter Fleischman was asleep, Raymond Dreyer staring, for some reason, over his right shoulder. The rest of us were riveted, dumbstruck, vacillating, I think, between fear for ourselves and awe at what we'd heard. It was Charlie White who finally broke the silence.

"Jesus Christ," he said. "You've been through it all, haven't you?"

George smiled. "Well, it's not so bad. When you think of it, all these things happen to everybody at some time in their life, only with me they happened all together. What's the big deal if your kid is born a bit wacky and your parents die? And hell, doesn't everyone have trouble with his brain?"

4

Managing Power

Surgery defined Brockman's day as the game defines the day of an athlete. No matter how routine the operation or how dramatic the events surrounding it, nothing competed with the time loop, the time-out-of-time that began when he entered the operating room and concluded when he took the elevator upstairs to the ninth floor to tell the family what he'd found. Operations were his theater, his prayer meeting, the consummation, emotional and sexual, of the romance that energized his life. He would tell you that no matter what his psychological state on the day of the operation, he left it behind when he entered the O.R. He would tell you—as others here would tell you too—that there was no time in the room, no distraction, no hunger. Though one stood almost all the time and leaned at awkward angles, fingers gripping instruments with force, ten or twelve or even fifteen hours could pass without muscular strain or fatigue. For some, like Benny Richmond, the O.R. was danger, risk, the exhilaration of high adventure, but for others who'd been around longer, like George Ahmad, the specialist in spinal surgery, the exhilaration had become so refined over the years that it was articulated in spiritual or (since Ahmad was a sculptor by avocation) aesthetic terms.

"Of course one gets high, but the high that used to come out of fear and danger is now, for me at least, a function of concentration, the absolute, almost lunatic attention one focuses. Now the excitement seems to increase as the operation proceeds. The nervous system is so elastic and deceptive that even the simplest disk will surprise me and teach me something. That's what turns me on. It's like sculpture in the sense that it requires terrifically subtle communication between one's hands and one's intuition, but unlike sculpture, of course, there is danger and the ultimate reason for the work, the patient's suffering, and your attempt to relieve it. When you combine all this, the risk and the learning and the concentration, the presence of death and physical pain, the possibility of healing, you get a situation in which you can't help but lose yourself entirely. And when you realize that—realize, I mean, that you've been standing there over the patient for twelve or thirteen hours without the slightest awareness of yourself —the whole process becomes religious. It's like you've left the human realm entirely."

Brockman would not dispute Ahmad's assessment, but he spoke of his work in other terms. Whenever he discussed surgery, two themes appeared and intertwined, primitivism and sexuality on the one hand, the "management of power" on the other. "Surgeons are interventionists, activists by nature, people who seek solution. Most physicians don't like an enforced decision-making process. Their problems go on in time, but surgical problems move very quickly toward resolution."

That was what he meant then by managing power: intervening in pathology, conquering matter and its perversity, conquering in effect Time itself—and therefore death. Unspoken though it was, this was the surgeon's dream. Brockman could sound callous at times, even vulgar, but there was a paradoxical vision behind the role he played, a great sense of the beauty of his work on the one hand, the arrogance on the other. If you listened to him long enough, he'd always come full circle. What after all was "taking problems out of time" except reaching for immortality? And what was immortality except the ultimate fantasy of power? And what was sex if it was driven, as he so often confessed, by the same conglomerate need? And how could it be denied if that was what it was? And how could it be accepted? If people like Ahmad articulated the process on higher planes, Brockman's point of view was as earthy and concrete—and finally as true—as the operating room itself. "There aren't many times I leave the room without at least a quarter of an erection. Hell, why not? It's all totally primitive, isn't it? You're dealing with danger, blood, power, conquering the man or woman on the table. No wonder wives of patients fall in love with surgeons. Aren't we the male who conquers her male? I tell you, the man who says he isn't turned on by surgery is either a liar or a eunuch or both."

If such statements seem melodramatic, consider the treatment of aneurysms, an operation Brockman and his staff performed forty or fifty times a year. The idea was to place a small stainless-steel clip on the root of the swelling, seal off the weak link in the artery, close up the patient, and leave the clip inside his brain forever. Imagine a weakness in the wall of a balloon, the air pressure causing a tiny teat to form on the surface, and then imagine the logical corrective, sealing off the teat at its root. The balloon wall in the case of aneurysms was the skin of the blood vessel. The pressure of the blood that flowed within the vessel was tremendous, and the aneurysm was often deep in the patient's brain, visible only through the operating microscope. The clip was inserted with a long microinstrument designed especially for that purpose. It had a spring on its tip which held the clip open, and a release mechanism on the other end which permitted the surgeon, when he judged the clip to be lined up just so with the base of the aneurysm and the surface of the blood vessel, to snap it into place. If the angle was wrong or the depth perception incorrect, if the instrument moved even a fraction of a millimeter when the spring was released, or if everything one did was correct but the base of the teat could not withstand the pressure, the vessel burst and the patient could die or suffer permanent neurological damage.* "Like a water hose in a plate of spaghetti" was how Brockman described the hemorrhage.

Current aneurysm therapy as practiced at Osler Memorial called for a two-week waiting period after the first hemorrhage, during which time the patient was maintained and sedated on a combination of drugs. It was estimated that of all such hemorrhages, 30 percent caused death at once. Among the 70 percent of patients who survived and were treated in this manner, 4 percent died during the waiting period, and the mortality-morbidity rate for the rest was 6 percent. The operation itself was no longer considered a significant risk. What they did was open the brain and spread it along certain established but —all brains being different and, as Ahmad said, elastic— always unpredictable pathways with an instrument called a brain retractor until, if they were correct in their maps and their reading of the angiograms, the aneurysm came into view. Then the clipping instrument was moved slowly into position, the clip sprung tight at the end, and, of course, the final moment when the clip was released, no matter how much preparation, knowledge, or experience was brought to bear on it, was pure judgment and instinct, grace under pressure if ever it existed. "Motherfucker!"

---

* In recent years, antihypotensive drugs have diminished this risk. Although it is estimated that 20 percent of aneurysms bleed during surgery, the bleeding is usually manageable if the blood pressure is lowered sufficiently. Some neurosurgeons use hypothermia as well to accomplish this purpose.

Brockman cried, the first time I saw him do it. "My pulse jumped fifteen points."

But when he left the room that day and the residents were, as they put it, "closing up" (he never did the routine work, opening and closing), when enough silence had been permitted to express sufficient respect for the man who was, after all, their guru, and the time arrived as it always did when he must be brought into human focus, the chief resident said to no one in particular, "He thrives on aneurysms the way Dracula thrived on blood."

Of course, Brockman was aware of the dangers contained within this mess of contradiction. "Surgeons who need to prove how big their cock is, they're the monsters of the operating room. Especially these days, when the measure of neurosurgical manhood is how much tumor you can get. You can't always distinguish tumor tissue from normal brain, so often when you think you're carving out tumor, you're actually digging into a patient's brain. Imagine how dangerous the guy is who has to get every piece of every tumor he encounters."

And sometimes it wasn't a question of how much tumor to take but whether to go after it at all. "We always say, 'If you want a conservative surgeon, find a busy one.' Because those who aren't busy are often so anxious to work—not so much for monetary as for ego reasons—so hungry for action, that their judgment can be distorted. When I was an attending, at the hospital where I trained before I came here, I was terribly frustrated because they wouldn't let me do any research or administrative work. I felt like I was burning up inside. During the last year it got so bad I couldn't stop operating. I did three hundred and fifty majors in that period, three hundred and fifty majors in one year, wouldn't let any of the younger people get the work they needed. Can you imagine how glad they were to see me go?"

———— · ● · ————

The surgeons' locker room was just down the hall from
the massive swinging doors (actuated by a button so that
nurses pushing stretchers or beds could open them) that
led to the operating rooms. Brockman had begun the day,
as he often did, in radiology, studying angiograms and
myelograms, until the chief scrub nurse phoned him to say
that the patient on the table was twenty minutes away
from ready, and we had hurried off to the O.R., winding
our way through the radiology department, which was like
a quick census of the current patient population, forty
people, at least, between the viewing rooms and the elevators, several waiting for chest or some other diagnostic
X-ray, some with broken arms or legs, stretcher cases with
I.V. bottles suspended above their heads, five wheelchairs,
two infants outside the CAT-scan room.

Near the elevator, we made one quick stop that morning
to say good-bye to Beecham, and while we were there,
Brockman delivered himself of what seemed to me the
perfect description of the dialectic I was presently exploring, the ridiculous contrast between his mind and my own,
surgeon-mind vs. writer-mind, the one absolutely concrete
and the other, until now at least, almost circumscribed by
abstraction. What, to put it bluntly, did the neurosurgeon
think of art? It wasn't necessary, of course, to generalize
from his response. In addition to Ahmad, who went to his
sculpture as soon as he left the hospital, Harvey Kellogg
played the cello, and both he and Beck were serious collec-
tors of contemporary painting. There was all sorts of extracurricular activity among the neurosurgeons which
was aimed at countering the narrowness of mind that
could accrue from the demands and influence of their
work. But still, as an example of the old school, the Boss
would suffice. Certainly the opinion here conveyed was
neither atypical nor surprising, nor—for that matter—remarkably different from those expressed by his younger
colleagues. It was Kellogg, after all, who once said to a
medical student who complained of feeling queasy during

neurosurgery, "Why? Do you feel queasy when you look
under the hood of a car?"

Having learned from the Boss, it was inevitable that
they'd develop sensibilities like his. And what was that
sensibility? Leaning over to pick up Beecham's desk
lighter (his last cigarette now before the O.R., his thirteenth of the day at ten fifteen), Brockman spied a piece
of orange pottery that looked to be broken from a pot.

"What's that?" he asked.

"Pottery," Beecham replied. "My wife's a potter, you
know. She's been trying to teach me how to glaze."

Brockman fixed his eyes on Beecham as if waiting for a
fuller explanation. When he saw that nothing more was
coming, he delivered what I'll always remember as the
ultimate expression of the priorities that exist within a
perfectly concrete mind: "Didn't you ever go to kindergar-
ten?"

Several surgeons were in the locker room when we arrived, and all of them were gathered around Harvey Kellogg, who had just finished a minor procedure. A forty-
one-year-old who specialized in vascular surgery and anastomosis, Harvey had recently returned from Switzerland,
where he'd purchased a new set of microsurgical instruments manufactured, according to his specifications, by
Swiss watchmakers. Seven instruments, stainless steel,
twelve hundred dollars. As he removed them from their
plastic wrapping, the crowd around him was not unlike the
one that might gather around a tennis player who showed
up in the locker room with a new racket, a runner with a
pair of shoes just come on the market. Everyone wanted
to hold them, touch them, shift them from hand to hand,
lift them to the light and squint along their edges as if
aiming rifles at the wall. Each instrument was eight to ten
inches long and honed to the minuscule tip that microsurgery requires, tiny scissors on one, a tweezer on another, a
knife on another. The needle holder—used for suturing the

tiny blood vessels that are severed and transplanted in an anastomosis—was capable of holding a curved micro-needle two millimeters long, and that needle would be threaded with nylon microsuture material a fifth as thick as a human hair.

These instruments were the products of microsurgical techniques developed in the late 1960s by M. Gazi Yazargil, in Zurich, and refined by biomechanical research recently initiated by neurosurgeons, who had realized that they were using instruments that had not changed a great deal since the last decade of the nineteenth century. Many, Brockman included, believed the work in this area had just begun. The instruments, in their view, were still not perfectly balanced or easy to handle. When I took them in hand myself, not being aware of their function or their defects, my appreciation was purely aesthetic, but that in itself was considerable. They were sensual in a perfectly negative sense, cold to the touch and the color of ice, their weight bespeaking remarkable density and compression. Holding them, I remembered Benny's search through philosophy and psychiatry and neurology and for a moment saw them as ultimate weapons against abstraction, a means by which one could penetrate thought and return to the source, the fundamental ground from which the whole miasma had emerged. For sure, it was impossible to touch them without wanting to use them at once. Or without remembering Brockman's allusions to sexuality and power. To "power, danger, and blood" they added all the contradictions of technology. Think of the bridge the aneurysm tool formed, the concrete channel between one man's brain and another's, imagine Brockman's finger and thumb—controlled by the motor strip in his own brain—manipulating it so as to release a clip in the motor strip of another brain. Correctly used, this instrument could save a leg, an arm, or a life. Misused or abused, it could, like any other tool, like technology itself, destroy all it meant to save. What was surgery after all but an ultimate expression of technology? And what was technology but an expression of the need to "manage power"?

Above us in the locker room was a loudspeaker, and a few minutes after we arrived, a woman's voice came over it. "Dr. Brockman, ready for you in surgery."

From a shelf near the lockers we took the green pants and shirts and the paper caps that everyone wore for surgery, dressed quickly, and hurried down the hall to the O.R. Across from Room 10, where the Boss always worked, we stopped in the washroom to scrub and put on our masks, but while I followed the carefully detailed steps on the sheet that hung over the sink—"Each fingernail should be stroked fifty times. Each stroke requires two motions. Each finger has four sides. Fingertips should be kept higher than the elbows"—he washed quickly and took the scrub sponge with him into the O.R. He was still washing (suds dripping onto the floor) when, a moment later, I hurried in behind him.

There was no easy way to discern that what I saw before me was a human being. Since neurosurgical patients are carefully draped (plastic, transparent drapes were tried once, but surgeons found it impossible to work if they could see the patient's face) so that only the exposed area of their brain shows, what I saw was a pulsating spherical object the color of watermelon streaked with gray and the texture (I guessed) of Jell-O. It might have been an arm, a leg, a stomach, or a part of an animal, and it might have been a piece of some exotic fruit. I knew it was a brain, but there was no way to relate the object before me to the connotations that word had come to generate in my mind. As the surgeons had promised, it was an object, nothing more, alive, to be sure, but a little absurd in its banality. During every operation I attended, there were moments when I had to remind myself that the organ I

saw before me was like the organ which which I perceived it.

Brockman introduced me around the room and eyes
flashed in my direction over masks. Thus commenced—
since I fixed my eyes on the nurses—a bit of the sexual
drama he had promised. There is nothing like covering the
face below the eyes to make one's dream of it seductive.
Great love affairs go on in surgery, and they aren't compromised in the least by the fact that lovers may not recognize each other if they meet outside the operating room.
Quickly, the almond eyes of the scrub nurse, who stood
like a conductor on the instrument stand above the table,
became my resting place, the world to which I turned when
the patient became unbearable. And if by chance I found
her looking back at me, I felt safe for a moment, secure
in the belief that, unlike the patient, I could not be dismantled.

The room was eighteen feet square with black-tile floor
and walls the color of eggshells. Huge kettle-shaped surgical lights, suspended from the ceiling, lit up the scene like
a movie set. No windows, of course, no odors except those
of chemicals in use, no sound beyond the sounds of surgery: the beep of the oscilloscope, the sighs of the respirator, the muffled commands of Brockman and his residents.
Insulation, as expected, was complete. On the wall facing
me was a large television set where the brain of the patient
was now displayed in living color. This was a recent innovation. The huge surgical microscope, also recent, was
attached to a TV camera (and a 35mm camera for taking
slides) which constantly displayed the view that surgeons
enjoyed on their field of operation. As a teaching aid, of
course, television is a godsend. No longer do students have
to crowd against each other, standing on tiptoes to look
over surgeons' shoulders. More important, when something interesting happens, they tape it, and the library of
tapes is always available to residents. Considering that

most neurosurgical technique, before TV, was learned on the job (though some was acquired from cadavers or animals), and that most residents therefore had to depend on the variety of patients who happened to come their way, the videotape has become a significant adjunct of surgical technique.

The set that hung on the wall was an ordinary TV. The image of the brain was bigger and brighter and soggier than the real one which could be seen over the Boss's shoulders, a bit more dramatic and maybe a bit less banal. Though events portrayed on the screen were simultaneous, of course, I found that I preferred the screen's version to reality, just as I generally preferred images of things to things themselves. Idly, looking over Brockman's shoulder, I inquired into the neurology of this particular phenomenon. What occurred in one's brain when the image replaced reality? Did the secondary image occur in one part of the visual cortex and the "real" image in another? The O.R. was not the place for such questions—which were, after all, the problems of perception (What is real and what is illusion? Is there truth beyond that which one perceives?) that have dogged philosophers for centuries—but it was not the place to avoid them either. Every once in a while they'd come upon me and distract me from the operation. It was fear, I think, that brought them on. I had expected that what I saw before me now would make me ill. And it was ever so much more convenient to think about philosophy than faint or vomit on the floor. What about the neurology of that? Does abstraction protect us from those responses in other regions of our brain (the middle ear, for one) which make us nauseated?

The patient today was supposed to be Charlie White, but he'd come down with the flu yesterday and they had sent him home to recover. In his place lay a ten-year-old boy named Billy Eggleston who had a tumor in his thalamus, an area deep, deep toward the center of the brain, just above the point where it joins the brain stem. If the X-rays were correct (and where this region is concerned it's not so easy to be sure), the tumor was just to the left and rear —ventral and posterior, as they say—of the pineal body, the point above the brain stem which Descartes called "the seat of consciousness." Not so many years ago, Billy Eggleston would have been sent home as inoperable, but the techniques of microsurgery have made it possible to go after tumors like this when the patient is young enough to justify the tremendous risk involved. Among other things, the brain stem contains most of the breathing centers. When the brain retractor gets down here and starts to move tissue around, the margins of error, if they exist at all, are infinitesimal.

Neurologists used to laugh at Descartes, but they don't any more. No one knows whether the mind is located within the brain, no one in all likelihood will ever know, but there's not much doubt that if it is, if "mind" can be materialized, it is most likely in the brain stem, the oldest part of the brain in terms of evolution, the one we share with animals. Within the brain stem there is a tiny tangle of neurons called the reticular formation, which extends from the top of the spinal cord up into the thalamus, connecting a number of direct routes with the "higher" cortical regions above it and the spinal cord below. Experiments with animals have convincingly established the reticular formation as the center of attention and awareness. Animals with experimental lesions confined to this region will be stuporous or comatose, and animals with electrical stimulators implanted here will learn much faster when the current is on than when it is off.

These experiments may account for the fact that there were more visitors than usual in the O.R. that morning, but the main attraction in all likelihood was the depth of the tumor and the delicacy of the approach that it required.

Of all regions of the brain that surgeons regularly treat, only one other, the pituitary gland, is as deep as this, and nowadays they go at pituitary tumors through the mouth, cutting directly through the gums.

The Boss was pleased at first with the residents' preparations. "Good job. Looks good, fellas," he said, but then suddenly he was angry. Noticing that a part of the flap had been left uncovered, he said, "Listen, you guys, why don't you act like surgeons? Put a piece of gauze over the midline, for Christ's sake. Shit, you're working on one place while the rest of that flap bleeds all over the floor." He turned to the anesthesiologist. "How much blood's he lost? Two units? Did you lower his pressure? Why not? Well, why not, for Christ's sake? He's a healthy young kid. You want to kill him?"

Throughout this tirade a nurse was helping Brockman into the last layers of his clothing, the surgical gown and the dark-brown skintight rubber gloves which, since they must be antiseptic, could not be donned until he entered the O.R., and finally the headlight that clamped on his forehead like a miner's lamp and connected to a transformer on the floor via a cord which ran down his back beneath his gown and trailed out from his rump like a tail.

When everything was in order and his anger burned out, Brockman touched Billy's brain in several places with his thumb, a gesture that shocked me. It looked as if he were poking about absentmindedly until he decided what to do. Later, Harvey Kellogg explained that all surgeons do it. "Before the turn of the century," he said, "surgeons used the finger irresponsibly, caused all sorts of fatalities with it, so it got a bad name. But there are things you can do with your finger that you can't do any other way. Separate the scalp from the skull bone, for instance, or palpate the surface of the brain"—that's what Brockman was doing now—"to find out the density of the subcortical tissue.

Sometimes the only way to stop a surface hemorrhage is with finger pressure."

The residents had opened the brain to the dura, which is the first (moving from the scalp toward the brain) of three fibrous membranes, the meninges, that separate the skull from the brain. (It is in this region that meningitis and tumors like Charlie White's occur.) With a tiny pair of scissors, Brockman now opened the dura. Since the meninges are interlaced with blood vessels, each cut produced trickles of blood like lines on a map, but Ed Jonas, the resident on Brockman's left, dabbed the blood away with cotton gauze and an electrically activated suction device, and Tony Reed, the resident on his right, coagulated the tiny vessels with an electrical tool called a hyphercator. Each time the hyphercator was applied it smoked and made a sound like bacon sizzling in a pan, and soon the foul smell of burning skin filtered through the room. Six hands moved along the surface of the brain, often colliding, bending around and sliding underneath one another. Gradually the opening in the dura took on nearly the same shape as the opening made in the skull, and when it was complete, the Boss drew the dura back onto a piece of moist cotton, or "Cottonoid" (one of their most important tools), bringing the brain itself into view. Then he laid another piece of Cottonoid on top of it and secured it with an automatic brain retractor that was clamped onto the base of the skull and held in place by a spring.

Their use of retractors was particularly ingenious when it was required that they be stationary. Hand-held brain retractors (which Brockman preferred) were bent to shape and edged around the tissue, and could be held in place with improvised clamps. The automatic retractors, though easily secured, often got in the way of other instruments and had to be readjusted. When retractors slipped, all hell broke loose, especially if the Boss was operating. Sometimes he stamped his foot like an angry child (a gesture that made a racket in the O.R. because like many surgeons he wore clogs), and sometimes he screamed at everyone in the room, searching out scapegoats for what were, in fact, unavoidable situations.

Twelve people circulated in the room: the Boss and his two assistants, three visitors besides myself (one of whom, I would discover, was the infatuated female medical student I'd seen a few days before in the office), a senior anesthesiologist and his assistant, and three nurses, including the scrub with the almond eyes who towered above the table, and the chief nurse, a tyrant named Millie who had whispered to me when I first came in the room, "If you feel like you're gonna faint, go to the corner so you don't fall on the patient." After that she kept her eye on me and corrected everything I did. "Don't stand there. . . . Don't lean on the wall. . . . That chair is for the surgeons. . . . Watch the wire!" I decided to avoid her. When she went to one side of the room, I went to the other, and when she watched the Boss work over his shoulder, I watched him work on television. For some reason, she eventually decided I could be trusted. I found that out when she came over to me with a clean gown draped backward over her shoulders, turned around, backed in close, and whispered in a sweet, almost seductive voice, "Tie me?"

Since everyone wore the same clothes, the only way to tell men from women (unless breasts were large enough to assert themselves through bulky gowns) was by their headgear. Hair had to be covered, but while the men wore regular surgical caps that tied behind their necks, the nurses wore colorful scarves. One was bright orange with butterflies, and Millie's had her name on it in little blue balloons. I found the vanity incongruous at first—here in this room that attacked the very concept of appearance—but there were times when the scarves relieved me. Like eye contact with the nurses, the vanity was a quick reinforcement of all the mythology that surgery insulted.

Sometimes the scarves alone could remind me what cata-
clysmic anxiety it induced to see a human being disappear
before my eyes, but sometimes too, on a day for instance
when I was taking myself too seriously, the surgery
treated *that* disease as much as the patient's, and the
scarves were just the right absurdity to help my treatment
on its way.

"Somebody give me a stool," the Boss said.

"That one there," Millie said, pointing toward the one
beside me. "Slide it underneath him."

It was a leather bicycle-type seat on a chrome stand with
wheels, and I pushed it forward between his legs.

"Ow!" he cried. "What the fuck you trying to do, cas-
trate me?"

I hadn't noticed that the stand had a pedal at the bottom
for adjusting the height. Realizing it now, I reached for the
stool, but as I did, I touched his arm and, jerking away, he
dropped his brain retractor on the floor.

"Oh, Jesus, you've contaminated me."

That brought the operation to a halt while his gown was
stripped off and replaced and a new set of gloves was
pulled on over his old ones. Nobody said a word to me or
even glanced in my direction. Things like this aren't so rare
in surgery, but when they happen, events swallow them
very quickly. At the moment, I wasn't altogether certain
that I hadn't killed the patient, but the Boss never mentioned the incident. Probably, since he couldn't see my
face, he didn't know me from any other observer in the
room.

By now they were near the tumor, deep within Billy
Eggleston's brain. One retractor had been clamped into
position, spreading the two hemispheres of the brain apart
and exposing the approach they intended to take to the
thalamic region. Looking over the Boss's shoulder, I saw
a dark cylindrical hole getting deeper as a second retractor
was inserted, and then, when he started to use the micro-

scope, I saw some of the complexities within that darkness, the anterior cerebral artery that ran along the midline between the hemispheres and the corpus callosum which connected them. The corpus callosum is one of the nerve tracts between the hemispheres that, when severed, produce the famous "split brain" patients that Roger Sperry has written about, people in whom the right and left sides of the brain do not communicate, who will sometimes pull up their pants with their left hand and try to drop them with their right.

"That's pretty, isn't it?" the Boss said, referring to the view of the corpus callosum which had just materialized.

He had continued his monologue throughout the operation, much of it simply commands for the scrub nurse or the residents, requests for cauterization or instruments. "Bayonet, please . . . hyphercate . . . sucker . . . pituitary forceps . . . hyphercate . . . hyphercate . . . ah, let's see, what I need now is a nice, clean number ten sucker. . . ."

Now, however, as he prepared to cut the corpus callosum, he became bad-tempered and impatient, the way he always did when the risks increased. "Give me a smaller brain retractor. . . . No, shit, that's the same one . . . put it in my hand, will you? Damn it, baby, watch my hands . . . if I have to turn it, you've passed it wrong. . . . Ah, shit, the retractor's slipping. . . . What's wrong with you, Tony, you want me to throw you the fuck out of this room? . . . Get it in place and secure it, will you? . . . Once we go into that corpus callosum there's no backing out . . . we can't have it slipping . . . it will start bleeding and kill this kid." Sometimes the anger was self-important and melodramatic, as if he were trying to psyche himself and sharpen his own attention, but sometimes too it was inevitable. There were too many hands moving about within the brain, too many instruments and too many clamps, too many veins and vessels to permit anything more than transient organization.

As the corpus callosum was severed, everyone except the Boss became very quiet with the tension. He was working with a retractor in his right hand and a hyphercator in his left, but the anterior cerebral artery was in his way and he had no hands to move it, so he turned his anger on Ed Jonas, who was supposed to take care of things like that but had no extra hands himself. "Goddamn you, Eddie, come on, will you? Put your sucker down and help me! Do I have to tell you what to do after all this time? Help me! Help me! I'm gonna throw you the fuck out!"

They managed finally to move the artery and hold it out of the way with a large retractor and a strip of cottonoid, but when the Boss went in again, this time with a bayonet, he hit a rather large vein that sent a small geyser of blood —nothing serious—clear out of the brain cavity. A few drops landed on his shoes, and Tony Reed, who'd taken most of it on his cap, made the mistake of saying what a normal man might say in such a contretemps: "Oops!"

"Oops?" Brockman said. "Five years as a surgeon and you still say 'Oops!'? C'mon, Tony, straighten up. It's bad table manners."

Everyone in the room cracked up, the Boss included, and in the commotion one of the surgeons moved the microscope and lost its angle. You couldn't tell which one had done it, of course, since it had two sets of eyepieces and any movement against either of them would throw it out of line—way out of line: its magnifications ranged from six to forty diameters. Watching the TV screen, you'd see the whole thing go suddenly berserk, and it could take them as long as ten minutes to find their place again.

When they got oriented this time, the Boss said, "Okay. There's the thalamus. Let's get this on tape, then I'll give you a look in real life."

What he meant by "real life" was a view directly through the microscope, which he offered to all of us who were visiting. When my turn came, I couldn't really find the thalamus in the tangle that looked something like spaghetti in aspic, but I said I did because it rather disoriented me to have the scope to myself, as if the brain and I were alone and it was looking back at me. This was one of the times when metaphor displaced reality in the operating room: the thalamus, after all, is the region of the brain in which all sensory experience is processed before being transmitted to the cortex. It was no small piece of ambiguity to confront it with one's own sensory apparatus.

When the female medical student got her chance with the scope, she asked what I suppose she thought was an intelligent question: "What's the chance this boy's gonna have binocular vision?"

"Oh, baby," Brockman replied, "you just flunked neuroanatomy. All that stuff's in the brain stem."

Retractors are thin, highly flexible instruments made of stainless steel. Surgeons shape them according to their eyeball estimate of the tissue they are about to encounter, and sometimes, after they get the tissue spread, they insert long pieces of Cottonoid to protect the passageway. The advantages of the Cottonoid, which looks as much like tape or gauze as cotton, are numerous. It is firm enough to spread tissue, soft enough not to harm it, and absorbent enough to draw off blood. Surgeons use it constantly as a protective buffer between instruments and tissue.

As the operation progressed, they were always severing veins or vessels, but unless they hit an artery or a tumor that was highly vascular, the bleeding seldom got out of hand. When it did, needless to say, problems multiplied rather quickly. General surgeons can use clips to stop bleeding, can even clip off an intestine, but clips are too dangerous for brain tissue and, if the bleeding is heavy, useless besides, because most of the time you can't see where the blood is coming from. What the neurosurgeons did in those cases was use the coagulator or the sucker, or both at once, trying to draw off enough blood to find the source and coagulate it.

Normal bleeding was controlled with an arsenal of coagulation equipment. Between the cottonoid and the suction tube, they were able to draw blood up almost as quickly as it appeared. In addition, they had several tools that coagulated electrically. When the tissue was fragile, they used the hyphercator, a tweezerlike instrument that passed a current through the tips; otherwise they used something called a Bovie forceps, which passed its current through the patient's body via a ground plate that had been placed beneath the buttocks before the operation began. There was also a Bovie loop, which cut and coagulated at the same time. One or the other of these instruments could seal off a blood vessel and stop most of the bleeding at once. In fact, the improvement in coagulation equipment was one of the principal reasons for the present low mortality rates in neurosurgery, and in general surgery as well.

With all the retractors secure and the microscope on target, they took a break to study the angiograms, which were posted on the wall behind them. One tends to forget that the world they were exploring is charted but roughly —the three and a half pounds of tissue packed within the skull so dense, with so much that is fragile and indispensable—and there's no way to know what's here or there, above or below, bigger or smaller, except from the angiograms and the CAT-scan, the latter a two-by-three Polaroid print and the former a twelve-by-fifteen negative, both two-dimensional shots of a dense, three-dimensional, asymmetrical sphere, difficult to read and very dangerous if one believes in them incautiously. You can see all these neat pictures in the neuroanatomy textbooks, the brain stem here and the pituitary gland there, the temporal lobe here and the frontal lobe there, but it's all approximation; no two brains are alike. It wasn't a large problem in an operation like this because the target area, though deep, was fairly easy to localize. When it got scary was when they were going through normal brain to get to a lesion or a tumor beneath it.

Once I saw them go after a tumor in the left temporal lobe of a ten-year-old girl, digging just about dead center in the dominant hemisphere, their instruments surrounded by regions that produce language and memory, soldiers dropped by night into a minefield.

"Won't that affect her language?" a student asked.

The surgeon shook his head and tapped the girl's brain with a retractor about four centimeters ahead of his incision. "No, language is up here."

When they went after tumors like that, they had to study the angiograms and CAT-scans very carefully and match them closely with what their incisions revealed, moving back and forth during surgery. But even then they had to follow certain road signs within the brain itself. "This is the vein that we see here on the angiogram . . . if we follow it, it will lead us to the vein of Galen . . . and unless we're not where we think we are, the vein of Galen when it moves from here to here is just about two centimeters above the tumor." Remember that for this girl they were cutting down into normal brain, not spreading brain apart as they did in Billy Eggleston's thalamic procedure but digging a hole in a dominant hemisphere and slicing tissue from the cavity. When they came in miraculously over the tumor, which was itself no more than one inch in diameter, located two inches beneath the dura, it was like finding gold, like an archer hitting the bull's-eye from a hundred yards in darkness. And more, much more miraculous, for the stakes were higher. If no one knew for sure precisely where the vein of Galen was, how the hell did anyone know that "language" was "here" instead of "there"?

While they were looking at Billy's X-rays, I took a walk around the room and for the first time saw the boy's feet. Bare, curling at the toes, and leaning sweetly against each other, they sent through me the greatest shock I'd felt since entering the O.R. It wasn't easy to derive personhood from the melon-shaped cavity at the other end, but this was different, and, as I would see time and again during surgery, nausea came only when one was reminded that the object on the table was a human being. Thus, the interior of the brain was rarely disturbing, but the skull as it was assembled or disassembled could send you reeling. Many times I went through an operation with equanimity but came near to dissolution when they reconstructed the patient's skull. So that's what it was! I'd think, leaning back against the wall. Sometimes, you see, you didn't even know what their angle was, whether they were operating on the left side or the right, the bottom of the skull or the top, and they were so clever about the sheet they draped around the patient, so good at cleaning up the blood, that the whole business, barring unforeseen events, was clean and even interesting. Put the skull back together, though, make it familiar, and watch the changes in your own brain when you make the right connections.

From the foot of the table I also got a better view of the technology that lay behind this sort of operation, the oscilloscope that gave readouts of the patient's pulse and blood pressure, the respirator that did his breathing for him (all muscles except the heart were immobilized before surgery), the equipment that collected and measured his urine, the drugs that increased or decreased his blood pressure and the pressure in his brain, the microscope, the camera, and the TV screen, the vault in the wall where their instruments were sterilized. It costs $200,000 to outfit a room like this today, and the portable equipment adds another $60–$70,000, the microscope and television another $7–$10,000. Considering that both a CAT-scan and an angiogram setup cost $500,000 and that postoperative care averages $500 per day, neurosurgery becomes a rather expensive trip to take. To me, it was one of the wonders of modern medicine that anyone, rich or poor, could be operated on by the Boss or his colleagues. They left it for the secretaries to handle bills and never knew themselves whether they had a welfare patient or a private patient on the table. Ken Beck estimated that 30 percent of his surgery was performed on paying patients. For the other 70 percent he collected nothing at all.

Ten minutes after they went back to work, one hour and fifteen minutes after the Boss had arrived and two and a half hours after the skull had been opened, they came to the tumor itself. As with the thalamus, Brockman gave us a view in "real life" and, as with the thalamus, I couldn't read anything from what I saw through the microscope. If tumor tissue differed from normal brain tissue, I couldn't see how.

In any event, as I stared into the scope, gazing down into a tunnel nearly two inches deep that ended at Billy Eggleston's brain stem, a medical student who had no doubt read the research on the reticular formation and accepted it as the solution to the brain-mind problem, whispered in my ear, "If there's a soul, man, you are looking at it."

"What I need now," said Brockman, "is a little copper spoon."

Since this was the part of the operation that would be most useful to residents, he kept the videotape running, explaining things as he went along.

"I'm scooping tumor now. There's a good view of the roof of the cyst. See, that's abnormal tissue. It's gelatinous. Like tapioca, I'd say. I don't know yet how much I can take, but it seems to have a pretty good capsule around it. From here it looks like a low-grade glioma. There's a chance this kid could live."

As the tumor was removed, they transferred it to a small glass for the pathologists, and when they thought they had enough, they took the rest with a sucker. It was very, very tricky down that deep, and great care had to be taken to cauterize the vessels ruptured so that no open wounds were left inside when Billy's skull was closed.

Several times the Boss cautioned the anesthesiologist to watch the pressure closely because he was pulling on the brain stem.

Finally he said, "I think that's about it," and withdrew his retractor. "I don't want to take any more." He stepped back and took off his headlamp, then his gloves. From the way he thanked the residents and the nurses, you'd never know there'd been any anger or confusion or missed instructions. It sounded as if they'd done their work perfectly, and for all I knew they had.

In the hall, Brockman walked toward the locker room with me and the female student trailing after him.

"That was beautiful," she said. "What an artist you are!"

He put his arm around her waist, opened the swinging doors, and let her pass before him. "Flattery," he said, "will get you everywhere."

In the locker room I asked him if the operation had been routine.

"No, oh no. That was pretty sexy. I haven't been down there more than ten times in my life."

He dropped one clog on the floor, sank into a chair beside the phone, lit a cigarette, and called the office. There was blood all over his gown and his pants.

"Hi, honey, it's me," he said. "Any calls?"

5

Origins

Although little is known about the intricate mechanics of a brain like Billy Eggleston's, a great deal is known about its origins. The first clearly discernible sign of the brain appears when the embryo in the womb is sixteen to twenty days old, about one twentieth of an inch in length. Prior to this, the fertilized egg develops into two hollow clumps of cells which are connected like a figure eight or the infinity symbol. At some point around the eighteenth day, this connection assumes a concave shape which embryologists call the neural groove. When the forward end of this groove thickens and expands, the evolution of the brain has begun. Slight swellings, already present, will become the eyes, the ears, and the nose. At twenty-five days, the groove has become a tube which begins to sink slowly toward the center of the embryo. The central cavity of this tube will eventually become the spinal cord, and its head end will become the ventricular system which washes the brain with the cerebrospinal fluid that nourishes it and protects it from shock.

Two types of cells, called neuroblasts and glioblasts, now begin to develop from the tube. They are the precursors of the glial cells and the neurons that will compose the brain. At this stage, neuroblasts can be extracted and kept alive *in vitro* for many generations, but at some point during their development into neurons, they will lose the capacity for cell division that, among other things, distinguishes them so radically from other cells. It is this incapacity which makes neurological damage, such as that which occurs in stroke, irreversible. If a portion of the liver or the skin is removed, the remaining cells will divide until the empty space is filled, but if a neuron dies, its space will be filled not with neurons but with glial cells, which do not possess, as neurons do, the ability to conduct neurological information. From the moment of conception to the moment of birth, an average of twenty thousand neurons are formed each minute, and when a child is born, it possesses almost all the ten billion neurons it will ever have. After birth, the only changes in neuron population will be negative, but although ten thousand neurons die every day, this amounts during a lifetime to only 3 percent of the total an individual possesses.

With the burst of cell growth, the various parts of the central nervous system begin to organize themselves into something approximate to their ultimate identities. The neural groove begins to turn into the spinal cord, and the first hint of the cerebral hemispheres becomes apparent in two bulges on either side of the tube. When the embryo is thirteen millimeters long, the tube thickens beyond the hindbrain to become the cerebellum, and two small bulges appear at the front. These, the optic cups, will develop retinae and connect via the optic nerve to the rest of the brain.

Changes now come quickly. "By the end of the third foetal month," writes Steven Rose in *The Conscious Brain*, "the cerebral and cerebellar hemispheres can be plainly traced, while the thalamus, hypothalamus and other nuclei can also be differentiated. In the following months the cerebral hemispheres swell and extend. By the fifth month the characteristic 'wrinkled' appearance of the cortex begins to develop."

The brain of the newborn child weighs 350 grams compared with the 1,300 to 1,500 grams of an average adult. It will be half its adult weight at six months, 60 percent at one year, 90 percent at six years, 95 percent at ten. For all this, however, the brain is closer to its adult state at birth than any other organ. It represents 10 percent of the entire body weight at birth and 2 percent at adulthood.

Physiological changes, measured by electroencephalogram, proceed apace with the biochemical. Very slow EEG waves can be detected in the third month of fetal life, but recognizable patterns do not occur until the sixth or seventh month. At twenty-eight weeks, volleys of so-called theta waves emerge, and at thirty weeks delta and alpha waves appear. Before thirty-two weeks, these waves are spasmodic, but the pattern then becomes consistent and the EEG can easily detect whether the infant is sleeping or awake. After birth the EEG pattern continues to change, and the ultimate adult pattern will emerge between the eleventh and fourteenth years.

Behavioral changes have continuously mirrored tissue growth. The heartbeat has commenced at three weeks and, as Dr. Rose notes, "an avoidance reaction—withdrawal of the hand-region by contraction of the neck muscles—occurs if an unpleasant stimulus is applied to the embryonic upper lip." At eleven weeks, swallowing movements will occur if the lip regions are touched, and at twenty-nine weeks there will be sucking movements and sounds. The whole range of behavior at birth, however, is reflexive, controlled mainly by the spinal cord and perhaps by some lower regions in the brain stem. While parts of the cortex are developed, it is not until after birth, when the child is confronted with an external environment, that true cortical behavior begins to emerge. After that, consciousness expands, and more and more of the individual's behavior comes under cortical control.

According to the *New Columbia Encyclopedia,* this three and one half pounds of tissue is "the site of emotions, memory, self-awareness, and thought." Such statements, as I've mentioned earlier, cannot be supported. Mostly, they are the result of pathological studies which demonstrate that a lesion in one area will produce predictable dysfunction, but this seems to me akin to asserting that I am in Kansas if, while you in California and I in New York are speaking long-distance on the telephone, the lines are cut in Topeka. To call this tissue the site of emotions, etc., is to call it "the mind," and that's a speculation which assumes a lot more than it can prove.

No one understands the wiring of the central nervous system. Some view the brain as a computer, and some as a holograph (with each specific cortical cell containing all the information possessed by the compendium). Some view memory as a function of particular regions, and some as a function of protein metabolism. (The latter theory in particular has gathered momentum lately; it is based on the fact that neurons are richer than any other cell in RNA, the huge molecules of which are capable of carrying inconceivable amounts of information.) Some view "mind" as a function of the reticular activating system, and some view it as an immaterial, universal continuum of energy that has nothing whatever to do with singular individuals. We know for sure that the wiring of the so-called higher functions involves the brain, but we don't know how. It is pure fantasy to derive from pathology specific topographic information on the mind.

What is not fantasy, however, is the power and mystery of this miraculous piece of pink and gray tissue, 85 percent water and the rest of it mostly fat, textured like oatmeal, shaped and wrinkled like a walnut, which in nine months evolves into an organ that makes possible the reading and writing of sentences like these; the motor dexterity and memory and judgment which allow one man to diagnose, say, an aneurysm, then cut into another's brain to seal it off; or the memory which permits storage of one million billion bits of information (more than the total stored in all the libraries and computers in the world), the control of sleeping and waking and body temperature and balance and appetite and growth, the experience of pain and pleasure, and the neurological understanding, recently emerged from research, that these contradictory sensations can often originate within the same bundles of cells. Typing and football, walking and riding, sex and laughter, rage and compassion and play and uptightness—none can be said to "originate" in the brain, but all can be eliminated forever if certain groups of cells are, through stroke or tumor or trauma, deprived of oxygen for three to five minutes. I may not be in Topeka, but if the wiring is defective there, we can forget about our conversation.

The brain is only one fiftieth of the mass of the body, but it uses one fourth of all the body's oxygen. Unlike the rest of the body, it has no storage capacity. It is entirely dependent on the blood flow for its glucose. Massive biochemical defense prevents its being used by the rest of the body as a food source, and this defense will withstand the threat of death from starvation. Like no other part of the body, it is without sensation (that's why neurosurgery is less painful than almost any other) and without immunity. It is, as they say, "immunologically incompetent." Is it ironic or simply logical that the center of our sensory and immunological systems should be itself without sensation and immunity?

Of all the brain's remarkable characteristics, the most striking may be its plasticity. It is not a static piece of tissue but a process, a transmitter as well as a receiver. The quality of its transmission is altered by what it receives, and the manner in which it receives is transformed

by what it transmits. It responds to and manipulates the
environment, responds to its own changes with more
changes. As we'll see, its chemistry and physiology, even
its anatomy, can change throughout a person's life. It is
affected by what we see, eat, feel, think, smell, or hear,
changed by music and literature and jokes and magnetic
fields, the quality of the air we breathe and the water we
drink, and, for all we know—since it is largely composed
of water and therefore susceptible to tidal pressure—by
the positions of the planets and the moon. A change in your
neurochemistry will make you love these lines or hate
them or find them incomprehensible, and if the lines are
good enough, they may themselves affect the status of
your brain. A concentrated brain is different from a distracted brain; concentration increases energy, neurochemistry can destroy concentration, concentration can control
neurochemistry, energy can produce concentration. Love
can change the brain, anger and sorrow can change it, and
neurochemistry can make us feel more loving, angry, or
sorrowful. In a fascinating experiment by C.R.B. Joyce,
two groups of ten people were isolated in different rooms.
In one, nine were given barbiturates and one ampheta-
mines, and in the other, the situation was reversed. "In
both rooms," Dr. Rose reports, "the 'odd man out' behaves
like his companions; the lone amphetamine taker behaves
as if he has been sedated, while the lone barbiturate taker
as if he has had sleep and fatigue abolished." The brain's
constant interaction with its environment is one of the
characteristics that make it so difficult to study, for among
other things it responds intensely to conditions in which it
is being observed. There are those who think that this fact,
more than any other, places an absolute limit on the extent
to which human beings will ever understand their own
brains, for the brain conscious of itself is fundamentally
different from the same brain when it is not.

These days I think most neuroscientists would agree

that the primary function of the central nervous system is inhibitory. From moment to moment we are bombarded with information from the outside world, the body, and the brain itself. The ordering principle sees to it that we are protected from the flood. The point where neurons meet (it is now known that they do not actually touch) is called the synapse, and the subtle, endlessly complex chemistry of the synapse is probably what determines whether an impulse moving along a neuron will stop there or continue to the neuron adjacent. There are neurochemicals which encourage the leap, and others which discourage it. A spectrum of chemicals is synthesized at the synapse, and their relative distributions may well determine a great deal of what we call our "state of mind." Some current theories of schizophrenia explain the disease in terms of an excess of certain chemicals which encourage synaptic exchange and/or an underproduction of those which inhibit it, the result being the overload of sensation which all of us know during periods of distraction but which those with "mental illness" experience almost all the time.

Presumably, if an impulse becomes an "awareness" or a "perception," it has somehow reached the reticular activating system and penetrated the selective net with which this region insulates and orders our perceptive functions. Consider that in the brain of a monkey each neuron makes ten thousand synapses with its neighbors. With ten billion neurons in the human brain, this would mean 10^{14} synapses in the cortex, or thirty thousand times as many as there are people in the world. Consider that neurons are firing all the time for a whole variety of reasons—and sometimes, it is said, for no reason at all!—and you get some idea of the explosion from which we are protected by the reticular activating system and the habituation function of the brain (those which prevent us, say, from feeling the shirt on our back more than a second or two after we've put it on; imagine our state of mind if we felt it, along with everything else, all the time).

For all the fact that these lower regions in the brain stem seem to control the "waking" functions such as awareness and perception, the "higher" functions like intelligence and consciousness are based in the so-called neocortex. This is the outermost layer of the cerebrum, the only area of the brain that has no equivalent in reptiles. In the earliest mammals it seems to have been concerned with motor behavior and coordination, but in higher mammals it develops great clusters of cells called association areas that are not wired to anything outside the cortex itself. Neurons here, says Dr. Rose, "talk only to one another and to other cortical neurons; they relate to the outside world only after several stages of neuronal mediation. ... In experimental animals whose association areas have been stripped off, there seems to be a learning deficit, although not always a straightforward one ... basic analysis of sensory input seems unimpaired." There is a steady increase in the size of the neocortex as the evolutionary ladder (as conceived, let us not forget, by the brains of human beings) is climbed, and in human beings the ratio of neocortex—and therefore association areas—to the rest of the brain is larger than in any other animal.

Obviously, not that any of us needs to be reminded of it, a great deal of space in our brains is available for argument and analysis, reflection, and reflection on reflection. Long after the brain achieves, in late adolescence, biochemical maturity, the association areas continue to change. In fact, present research indicates that these regions, unlike any others, may change as long as a person lives.

War exists within the brain (something else we don't need help to recall). Arthur Koestler, in his book *The Ghost in the Machine*, has laid a great deal of human misery to the conflict between the "new" brain and the "old," the so-called limbic brain we share with reptiles, which still controls our emotions, and the cortex, which controls our reasoning process. Much too has been written about the opposition between the left and right cerebral hemispheres, most of it the result of recent surgical procedure which has permitted, in cases of intractable brain damage, a severing of certain tissue (like the corpus callosum) that connects them. A great deal of simplistic neuropsychology has emerged from this research, most of it romanticizing the right hemisphere as the source of music and intuition and a host of other "integrative" functions, while the left is cast as the heavy—logical, verbal, and linear, the only barrier between us and perfect innocence. For all the banality of many such theories, left-right brain research is a rich vein that has only begun to be mined. Among other things (as Julian Jaynes reveals in *The Origin of Consciousness in the Breakdown of the Bicameral Mind*), it has provided a focus for new perspectives on the study of language and consciousness, certain distinctions and identifications between the two that have been suspected all along but now begin to be verified.

What's wondrous about the brain is the variety of ways in which it can be studied. Philosophers, psychologists, sociologists, theologians, mystics, and, of course, neuroscientists—among whom we could offer subcategories like neurochemists and neuropsychologists and neurophysiologists—all have their own particular systems in which the brain is as close to First Cause as one can get while remaining in the physical world. All these disciplines are revelatory and, in their own way, irrefutable. One can explain psychology in terms of chemistry or chemistry in terms of psychology, a belief in God in terms of neurophysiological propensity or neurophysiology in terms of a belief in God (which alters brain function, does it not?). If the driving need to articulate the causal chain of behavior is committed to the concrete world, the brain becomes the focus of almost any investigation, and its use will vary according to the language and the conceptual systems through which it is observed.

Of all such systems, however, only one offers a direct therapeutic modality, and that is neurosurgery. Limited though it be in its abstractions, it is the only means by which living human brains are observed directly by other brains—and minds—and from that point of view it is a perfect consummation of the brain's fascination with itself. When Wilder Penfield stimulated the brain of a conscious patient and produced a chain of memory, he was expressing an archetypal human dream: to derive from the body that which is not of the body, locate the source of nonmaterial experience in the world we know through our senses. The history of neurosurgery among other things is the history of this dream in its most primitive form.

Although neurosurgery as a science did not exist until the 1880s, archeologists have unearthed skulls two thousand years old—in Egypt, Greece, and Peru—which show proof of surgical entry. It is thought that these patients were treated for insanity, epileptic fits, or severe headache, the idea being to relieve symptoms by diminishing the brain's internal pressure. (It is not at all unlikely that such treatment succeeded. Very often, when the dura is opened, excess fluid or blood will drain and intracranial pressure diminish.) The anesthesia of choice was wine; the preferred antiseptic, honey. The surgical tool, a kind of circular saw-drill called a trepan, was used by neurosurgeons in an improved form (trephine) until the 1920s, and it is still used by certain primitive tribes. Most of the unearthed skulls were opened in the area above the so-called motor strip (where Charlie White's skull would be opened), but it is fairly certain that all entry stopped at the meninges, or outer layers, of the brain. Although a French surgeon, Baron Guillaume Dupuytren, reported in the early part of the nineteenth century that he had cured a patient completely by "thrusting a long knife" into the brain and causing "pus" to well up through the opening, it is thought that work within the brain itself was not risked until the late nineteenth century. Still, Hippocrates was a pretty good neurologist as well as a neurosurgeon. He knew in 300 B.C. that "a blow to one side of the head was sometimes followed by paralysis or convulsions on the other [side of the body]," and he recommended neurosurgery for blindness when there was no clear sign of eye disease.

Most of the knowledge gleaned by Hippocrates and other Greek physicians—like Claudius Galen, who is said to have been the first experimental neurologist—was preserved in Alexandrian libraries that were destroyed in wars during the early centuries after Christ. From this time until the appearance of such famous sixteenth-century anatomists as Vesalius and Fallopius, clinical medicine was almost completely stagnant. Although trepanning returned in the thirteenth century (wine still used as an anesthetic), it is generally accepted that there were no great advances in surgery until 1850. As for neurosurgery, knowledge of the physiology and anatomy of the central nervous system was insufficient to permit it on anything more than a rudimentary level until 1880.

At this time, three crucial developments set the stage for its advance. First, Joseph Lister's antiseptic techniques made it possible, for the first time, to offer surgical patients some safety from infection, and second, advances in anesthesiology brought about a radical reduction in the pain and terror that surgery produced. Finally, a series of brain localization experiments by such men as Hughlings Jackson (called by many the greatest of all neurologists) confirmed what had been suspected since the days of Hippocrates, that specific regions in the brain controlled motor and sensory response, while others were involved with language and memory. These days we take localization for granted, but the modern view of the brain was not accepted until the eighteenth century, not confirmed until the nineteenth. Aristotle, who thought that the mind was located in the heart, considered the brain's principal function to be something like an air conditioner's, cooling the blood that passed through it, and many scientists after him believed the liver to be the seat of emotion (Isaac Asimov suggests that this is where the term "lily-livered" originated).

The first modern neurosurgical procedure was performed in 1884 when Sir Rickman John Godlee, using Lister's new antiseptic techniques, removed a tumor localized by the new neurological methods. (The patient died, but of a fungus infection.) The father of modern neurosurgery is thought to be Sir William MacEwen, a Scottish surgeon who performed his first brain operation in 1876 on a dead patient. Although permission for the operation had been denied by the patient's parents, this was the first time a predicted lesion was verified concretely. Once this barrier was crossed, expansion was rapid and international. By 1886, Victor Horsley, an English surgeon, had done ten brain operations; by 1888, MacEwen had done twenty-one, with eighteen recoveries (needless to say, where neurosurgery is concerned, particularly the primitive neurosurgery then being performed, the concept of recovery must be taken rather loosely); and by 1890 neurosurgery had spread to Germany and the United States. The American pioneer was W. W. Keen of Philadelphia, one of whose early patients, reported well after thirty years, is considered the first neurosurgical case to produce unqualified cure.

During the next twenty years, support came from all directions. Neurological research—fired by a belief that total understanding of the central nervous system was imminent—moved into a period of feverish activity. Clinical technique became more scientific and rigorous, blood transfusion became feasible in the early 1900s and lumbar puncture in 1891, and the study of the ductless glands such as the thyroid, the thymus, and the pituitary became more focused after 1910. In 1918, the Baltimore surgeon W. E. Dandy made the first use of ventriculography—a method by which air is injected into the ventricles to permit observation by X-ray—and in the early 1920s, Harvey Cushing invented methods of electrocoagulation which made it possible to control all but the most extensive bleeding.

Great advances too had been made in techniques for opening the skull. Until the late nineteenth century, opening had been accomplished much as in the days of Hippocrates. A target area was outlined on the scalp, a hole drilled at the center by trephine, and, as described in E. Stephens Gurdjian's *Operative Neurosurgery*, "portions of bone were removed by means of large, bonebiting forceps." In the 1890s, an Italian named Francesco Durante made an incision in the shape of a horseshoe and then, with "power-driven, circular saws . . . and a gouge with a wooden hammer," cut along the sides of the horseshoe and left the base intact. Though simplified, this method of craniotomy, called an osteoplastic flap, is still in use today. The major problem after that was mechanical—how to cut through the incredibly hard bone without endangering the tissue beneath it. In 1909 W. H. Hudson, an American, developed a drill with spiral cutting blades and protective shoulders that resisted cutting when it reached the dura. Once the holes were drilled, the bone was either chopped away with forceps or cut from inside out with a Gigli saw —a flexible wire blade which was inserted through one burr hole and threaded between scalp and skull to a hole some distance away. All these refinements made the craniotomy more sophisticated, less traumatic, and less dangerous, but also slower. The procedure for brain tumor, which now requires four to ten hours, was once accomplished in sixty minutes: quick opening by trephine, quick tumor removal with spoon or finger, packs to control hemorrhage, and loose scalp sutures to permit drainage of spinal fluid. Nowadays, opening and closing require at least an hour before and after the critical stages of neurosurgery. Removal and reconstruction of the skull is routine and almost fail-safe, but it is also tedious and strenuous, as hard as any manual labor in the hospital.

Between 1889 and 1899, brain tumors were diagnosed only thirty-two times in thirty-six thousand patients admitted to Johns Hopkins Hospital in Baltimore. Of these thirty-two, thirteen were proposed for surgery, but only two, with fatal results for both, went to operation. By 1910, after practicing neurosurgery for a decade, problems remained in the control of hemorrhage and infection, Harvey Cushing alone had performed 250 operations.

Cushing's arrival on the scene was itself a crucial event in the history of neurosurgery. He was the first to devote full time to the specialty, a great innovator in the operating room, a brilliant clinician. If his biographers are correct, he was not only the clinical father but also the psychological antecedent of men like Brockman and Kellogg, the first clear example of the sort of personality that neurosurgery seems to attract and/or produce. Like Brockman's, his energy and volatility were legendary. He was said to be vicious with those who made mistakes and, even in his late sixties, almost unnaturally devoid of fatigue after surgery. Like Kellogg, he was an avid collector of medical histories, famous for his library and the articles derived from it, and like Wilder Penfield, he had a full-fledged literary ambition. In 1948 he produced a two-volume biography of Sir William Osler, the great internist, for whom Osler Memorial was named. The book won a Pulitzer Prize

and is considered one of the great classics of medical literature. He was an accomplished draftsman whose medical
sketches remained great teaching aids until the camera
became practical in the operating room, and he was a remarkable inventor; in addition to electrocoagulation equipment, he devised a number of tools and surgical aids that
are still in use today.

In a 1915 study, mortality rates for neurosurgeons' patients were compared for the first time. They ranged from
50 percent for Fedor Krause in Berlin to 8.4 percent for
Cushing. Cushing was said to have lost no patients to
meningitis, while others lost an average of 10 percent. But
again, such figures must be kept in perspective. As Brockman explained, "Cushing had a low rate because he didn't
do much. With acoustic tumors, for example, he'd remove
the center and leave the cyst intact. It's when you go for
the cyst that the risk increases, because that's where it's
attached to the brain." Cushing did not treat aneurysms,
and he would never have considered operation on a tumor
as deep as Billy Eggleston's. In fact, neurosurgery as
practiced by Brockman and his colleagues is as different
from that practiced by Cushing as Cushing's, at the end of
his career, was different from MacEwen's.

The great advances since Cushing have been diagnostic
and pharmacological. Drugs like mannitol have made it
possible to control both intracranial and blood pressure,
corticosteroids control the swelling of the brain after surgery (and sometimes, by inhibiting a tumor's swelling,
make surgery unnecessary), and of course, Dilantin and
phenobarbital have literally restored life to those who live
beneath the shadow of unpredictable seizure. For diagnosis, Cushing had no angiogram—that was invented by
Moniz in 1929—and there was no CAT-scan until 1973.
Brockman rarely did exploratory operations, but Cushing
did them all the time (he operated on one patient seventeen

times). Today, with such drugs protecting them and such foreknowledge provided to their surgeon, neurosurgical patients are at no greater risk statistically than ulcer or orthopedic patients. For sure, Brockman promises no picnic, but because of the drugs now available, the efficiency of techniques for opening and closing, and the remarkable advances in hypotensive anesthesia, a Cushing patient would probably consider neurosurgery today a sort of lark. What's more, many patients whom Cushing would have turned away are cured these days because the operating microscope—introduced by the Swedish ear, nose, and throat surgeon G. Holmgren in the early 1920s and modified for neurosurgery by Yazargil in the 1960s—provides access and instrument control where the human eye cannot. Add to this the teaching value of videotape, the preparation it provides a surgeon that was never before possible. If Cushing, as Brockman put it, "went in on the seat of his pants," today we can at the very least expect our neurosurgeons to meet us standing up.

What about the future? A great deal of surgery performed now may not be done at all in ten or fifteen years. Most people think that lethal brain cancers—gliomas, for example, like those which afflicted Raymond Dreyer and Peter Fleischman—will be treated by chemotherapy or radiation. It is also expected that embolization—the amazing technique by which catheters are introduced into major arteries, threaded to the brain under the guidance of angiography, then used as a conduit for glues or plastics or even small balloons which seal off aneurysms or arterial malformations—will make it possible to treat a good deal of vascular disease without incision. Another innovation, already much in use, is stereotaxis. Through precise measurement and guidance, needlelike instruments are inserted through tiny holes in the skull and then used for controlling spasticity or other physiological problems by freezing limited regions of the brain. Soon, it is expected, stereotactic instruments will be guided by computers linked to CAT-scans, and they will home in on minuscule areas (one centimeter out of fifty) in the thalamus to control tremors or seizures. Brockman expects that stereotactic surgery will replace seizure surgery such as that performed in Montreal on George Tinker and some think it may also prove effective in the treatment of tumors or intractable pain. Concerning the latter, I. S. Cooper and others are also experimenting with the implantation—usually in the cerebellum—of electrical stimulators (some of the newer versions programmed by telephone), and these too have shown great promise in the treatment of pain and tremors.

Ironically, much of this progress may work against neurosurgery. Mention has been made earlier of the overabundance of neurosurgeons in this country and the great danger they pose to a profession which, more and more, begs for centralization. The malpractice controversy and the crazy inflation of medical costs will restrict specialists like neurosurgeons more than others, and the more it does, the less likely it will be that they'll take the risks their work requires. Political issues will tend to favor low-cost medical treatment over sophisticated procedures like that performed on Billy Eggleston. Finally, there are the political and moral problems of psychosurgery, which surfaced in the 1940s when prefrontal lobotomies were performed with dispatch to control almost any behavior (depression or violence, for example) that made patients or others uncomfortable. Stereotaxis is already being used for treatment of such "disorders" as "violence" or "excessive sexuality," and the chances are high that the more efficient this technology becomes, the more it will be abused.

For all that, the neurosurgeons have come a long way since Cushing, not to mention Hippocrates. They'll never be able to help us—if I may paraphrase Charlie White—

get our heads in the right frame of mind, but there's a lot
better chance today that when our brains intrude beyond
the call of duty on the function of our minds, someone like
Brockman or Kellogg will be able to redress the balance
and send us off to our proper, if absurd, neurological deserts.

6

One Lovely Doctor

After operating on Billy Eggleston, Brockman took a
little time in the locker room to get himself together and
prepare for the outside world. One bare foot on the coffee
table, one still encased in his bloody clog, he smoked four
cigarettes, gossiped with other surgeons, and caught up
on his telephone calls.

"Martha, hi, this is Jim. We got the pathology on Mr.
Hickens. It's a primary brain cancer. . . . Yeah, we thought
it might be a metastasized melanoma, but we were wrong.
. . . Oh, sure. He's doing pretty well. We took him out of
the I.C.U. yesterday. . . . About a year, I'd say. Certainly
not more than fourteen, fifteen months. You know his
wife's dying, don't you? He's been awfully depressed
about that. . . . Sure. I'll say hello for you."

And then: "Tony, hi, how're you doing? Listen, I saw
your patient, what'sisname, Frankel? His wife's convinced
he's got more tone in his face, and he can drink now without drooling. Obviously that's encouraging, but it's still
too soon to say about the facial nerve. . . . What's that?
. . . Why not? He's got another six months before we write
it off."

I went across the hall and bought us coffee and sand-wiches from the cart that was stationed there to service O.R. personnel. Brockman took one bite of his tuna sand-wich and threw it in the trash can. "I can't eat after that kind of surgery. Shit, that kid wrung me out."

I asked what would have happened to Billy if there had been no operation.

"He'da been dead in three months."

"What about miracles? Did you ever see a tumor like his clear up for no good reason?"

"Never. It gets them all, sooner or later."

Awkward as ever with the telephone, he dialed another number very slowly. "Claire? Hi, honey. Anybody looking for me? . . . Yeah, sure. Tell him I'll be back in the office around twelve thirty. Listen, do me a favor, will you? Every pair of pants I own has a hole in the pocket. I'm losing everything. Can't you talk to those guys at the cleaners and get them to fix a pair for me? I've got nothing to wear for my talk tomorrow. . . . Mrs. Karallo? Shit, I forgot about her. Give me her number."

He dialed again without replacing the receiver. "Mrs. Karallo, hi, this is Dr. Brockman. How are you feeling today? Still nauseous? Are you dizzy too? Okay. We better get you in for another scan. Call my office and they'll make an appointment for you."

Hanging up, he turned to me. "Every fucking rinky-dink hospital has got to have a CAT-scan. Half a million dollars and they don't know how to use it. Shit, I knew her scan was no damn good the first time she brought it in. Mir-acles? Did I ever tell you about Barbara Zinn? When she was twenty years old, she went to a neurologist in Balti-more with memory loss and lethargy. He told her family she had a tumor and three months to live, and they hid it from her, told her she had encephalitis, assured her she'd be okay in two or three months. A few days later, she woke up and heard her sister crying in the bed next to her. She knew somehow that the sister was crying about her, and it came on her in a rush that they'd all been lying to her. 'I was dying,' she told me, 'and it was like they were conspiring to keep me out of my own death.' She was hurt, confused, and enraged, of course, and she didn't calm down until she went to a psychiatrist and he told her what they all assumed was the truth—inoperable cancer, three months to live. Then everything turned around. She took over the whole show, rallied the family around her, got everyone involved in preparations for her death. Then she came to me and I operated on her and found one small, metastatic nodule in her right frontal lobe. She made a complete recovery from the operation, and the search for the primary cancer proved negative. Now it's been five years since surgery, and she conducts herself as if she's permanently cured. She just graduated medical school and she's planning to go into neurology."

"Well," I said, "that's pretty close to a miracle, isn't it?"

"Maybe, maybe not. Last week, she came in with real bad headaches and blurred vision. We're doing a CAT-scan on her tomorrow."

While he took his shower, I sat back and took in the show of the locker room. Surgeons were coming and going all the time, some in street clothes to dress for the O.R., others in scrubs, returning from operations. Like locker rooms anywhere, this one was insular, safe from the outside world, aggressively communal. Conversation was small talk unless surgeons were from the same department. Then, sometimes, they would talk about what they had done or planned to do.

"How's the kid?"

"We got it, I think. We'll know in a while if he's breathing on his own."

There were two rooms, carpeted in green, with low ceilings, fluorescent lights, beige-colored metal lockers, shelves along one wall for scrub clothes, barrels for dirty clothes, a large trash can for disposable stuff like shoe covers, caps, and masks. A bulletin board on the wall displayed an advertisement for a charity ball, raising money for the hospital, and several personal notices, two people looking for summer places, one offering an apartment for sublease. Except for the loudspeaker which called surgeons from the O.R., there was no sound from outside the walls. In one corner, there were three small cubicles with gray telephones that connected to dictation equipment somewhere in the depths of the hospital, and surgeons used these to record their notes just after surgery. It was all very streamlined: within the hour the cassettes were delivered for typing to secretaries in the surgeon's office. As one would expect, it was no small piece of irony to hear "the power" and "the blood" and "the primitivism" reduced so quickly to techno-prose, intonations utterly devoid of emotion:

"Under adequate preoperative sedation, comma, general endotracheal anesthesia, comma, a line was placed in the right femoral artery, comma, a central venous pressure line was placed in the right femoral artery, comma, a central venous pressure line was placed in the right anticubital fossa and a large pore peripheral catheter was placed in the left forearm, period. The right iliac crest was prepared and draped in the usual manner for taking a bone graft and the patient was prepared and draped for an intracranial and extracranial hypertelorism and repair, period. A curvilinear, comma, anteriorly placed scalp flap was fashioned and a bifrontal coronal approach was used to expose the anterior portion of the cranial fossa, period."

Done with his shower, Brockman sat down in his underwear for another cigarette and another cup of coffee (he drank eight or more on an average day). I noticed a large ugly scar in the middle of his back.

"Skin cancer, last year," he explained. "I was supposed to go back to my surgeon's office to have the stitches taken out on Monday, but it looked good to me, so I got one of my boys to take them out on Friday afternoon. Next day I went fishing, had the boat out by myself, and hooked into a big bluefish. I was up on the bridge, but I shut down the engines and swung down to the deck to bring him in. Felt a twinge in my back but ignored it. Later, when I came home, my wife says, 'Hey, you're bleeding all over!' Jesus, there was blood all over my shirt and I hadn't even noticed. I went upstairs, took off my shirt, and looked over my shoulder in the mirror. Saw this big gaping wound, fat and muscle poking out, thought, Hey, that's me! and got nauseous as hell. That's the only time in my whole life when I've been nauseated at the sight of blood."

A few minutes later we went out to the elevator, heading upstairs to meet with Billy Eggleston's parents, who'd been waiting since early morning for the results of his surgery. Just opposite the elevators was the recovery room, where patients were taken when they left the O.R. and kept until they were more or less out of danger. To the left of the doorway two infants were screaming, and the only other patient I could see had tubes and arterial lines protruding from his body as if he were a machine not quite assembled. Nurses were busy here, constantly on guard for postoperative clots and hemorrhage. A radio on the desk was tuned to the local rock station, playing, at that moment, Linda Ronstadt's "Blue Bayou."

Kenneth Beck had operated on one of the babies, and we met him now as he came out of the recovery room. He was still in his scrub suit, about to begin on another child, but he paused for a rather frigid conversation with the Boss.

"I'm sorry about that stuff, Ken."

"Well, it's not right. It's not the way things ought to work around here."

"I know. But this time it couldn't be helped. They were stubborn as hell."

"We run the hospital, not them."

"Yeah, sure. You're right. Let's hope it doesn't happen again."

Waiting for the elevator, Brockman explained that Beck was angry because he had operated on Billy Eggleston when he, Beck, was supposed to handle pediatric cases. Things like this happened all the time because the Boss was the big name here, and people who had been referred almost always wanted him. It made no difference to them that Beck might be better at pediatrics or that Kellogg was one of the best in the world at anastomoses. It was Brockman's name that made them feel secure, and if he tried to pass them on, they would often feel shortchanged. It was a problem common to teaching hospitals, serious not only because it bruised egos but also because it slowed the development of younger people by depriving them of experience. This time, however, since Beck had all the work he could handle, it was only an ego problem, one which, as it turned out, would be rectified in a few days.

"Fortunately," Brockman said, "Ken's got a better case tomorrow. His will be the star at Friday conference, not mine."

All sorts of politics got juggled in the hospital. Departments, as I've mentioned, often butted heads, neurology against neurosurgery, cardiology against internal medicine, orthopedics against rheumatology. When you wanted a language test for an aphasiac, did you call the aphasia specialist from the psychiatry department or one of the speech pathologists from rehabilitation? Clinical psychologists were patronized by psychiatrists, and social workers by both, nurses aides by nurses, lab technicians by pathologists. On a given day, war could break out between administration and the staff, between both and the directors of government insurance programs, between all three and community groups seeking better care for the poor.

As chairman of the medical board (the governing body of the hospital), Brockman was at the center of it all, hatch-ing a plan, for example, to withhold the paychecks of residents who did not complete their patient charts and feeling out the union to see if they'd permit it. He loved these machinations. There were those who thought that administration and medical politics interested him more at this point in his career than surgery, but they were wrong. It was all "management of power." The super joys of intervention came in every size and shape.

His major problem now was a complex struggle between the staff and the management arm of the hospital, called the General Hospital Corporation. The staff had been working with the union to develop a medical-insurance plan for hospital workers, including themselves, but it had lately come to their attention that the corporation—hypersensitive because of all the publicity about runaway medical costs—had literally planted spies all over the hospital to report on staff performance. A confrontation was brewing, the corporation denying the espionage and the staff becoming more and more suspicious. ("How can we work on an insurance plan," said one, "if they're knifing us in the back?") So Brockman had dug into his own political pocket and called up an old friend, a fishing partner, who happened to be head of one of the largest unions in town, pals with both the boss of the hospital workers union and the chairman of the corporation. "If this guy works for us," he said, "they won't stand a chance."

Federal money was politics too. Without it, you could forget research, and without research you could forget the reputation of your department. At this point the neurosurgical department's research budget was $1.25 million a year, but the stakes were about to increase dramatically. Applications had been filed for a spinal cord grant of $5 million and a head-trauma grant of $3 million (both to be spread over five years), and you could be sure that the success or failure of the submissions would depend not only on Brockman's clinical skill but also on his connections and timing and political sophistication. The head-trauma grant in particular would put him to the test. The proposed program would take patients with catastrophic head injury and—after all other treatment had failed—hibernate them for three or four days at flat EEGs, holding their brain waves as near to zero as possible while still keeping them alive, and then bring them up again and see what effect this had on their mortality rates.

Although the idea was sound and not unprecedented, and Osler had the staff and facilities and patients (who were often brought in by helicopter to a heliport adjacent to the hospital) to make such a program work, the head-trauma application, at this point, stood a good chance of being rejected. On grants of this size, the National Institutes of Health (N.I.H.) sent out an observation team to study the clinical and laboratory environments and interview those who would direct the project; it would then report back to the board of trustees, who made the final decisions. This team was committed to secrecy, but if like Brockman you happened to be friends with one of its members, you could often find out how things were going. If the team was leaning against you, you could make some adjustments and, if you had the confidence of the trustees, request another team before the final decision was reached. In the case of the head-trauma application, a friend of Brockman's had confided that the team thought the number of patients involved—only twenty a year at a maximum—made the program what the N.I.H. called a "feasibility study" rather than the large-scale, random, statistical research they thought necessary to justify a $3-million grant. Three times that week, Brockman had been on the phone with friends in Washington, pleading his case and seeking another team he hoped would be more sympathetic.

What made the process especially difficult was that, even if the money was obtained, the application had to be updated in eighteen months and was subject then to revocation. This meant that all the people hired with the money —the basic scientists, neurosurgeons, neurologists, anesthesiologists, technicians, and physical therapists who made such research possible—could not feel secure in their appointments. The greatest problem for those in charge of big research facilities like this was keeping the good people away from the big money and security available to them in industrial laboratories. And here at Osler the deciding factor, what made them take the risk and stay, was very often the Boss's reputation and the political clout he was thought to have. Was it any wonder that those who would choose Brockman's successor, after he retired, would have to look for a lot more than clinical and surgical skills?

José Rivera was on the elevator when it came, and he and the Boss got down to business. There was talk about an intern who had just "rotated" through the department, Brockman seeking José's opinion as to how he should be graded—"He did what he had to do, but nothing more," José said; "his girl friend was giving him trouble"—and then consultation about an eleven-year-old girl who had hemorrhaged after surgery two days before and had gone back to the O.R. at three that morning. José wanted the Boss to look at her in the I.C.U., and he promised to do so when he was done with Billy Eggleston's parents. At the pediatric floor, José got off and Harvey Kellogg got on, and during the course of the two-floor ride between pediatrics and adult neurosurgery they conferred about Victor Alfredo and his giant aneurysm.

It was like this all day, every day. Brockman was seldom alone when at large in the hospital, almost never not working. The elevators and halls were extensions of his office, and the door of his office was never closed except for very special meetings. In fact, the department seemed to be devoid of concern for privacy. It was an accepted practice that anyone, including me, could not only use Brockman's office while he was gone but look through his desk for books or letters or anything else required at that particular moment. Since he came to work as soon as his morning exercise was done (eating breakfast in the cafeteria) and did not go home until he was ready for bed, the line between his public and his private life was almost nonexistent.

We got off at the ninth floor, and as Harvey hurried down the hall, two women converged on Brockman from opposite directions: Raymond Dreyer's daughter and Andy March's wife. He got rid of them both by promising to see them later, during evening rounds, but before he got to Billy's parents, who were sitting by the window in the Visitors' Lounge, he had to deal with the chief nurse, who had an equipment problem, and then with David Getz, who had heard the Boss's voice from his tiny office adjoining the lounge and wanted to discuss a newly admitted patient, a nineteen-year-old quadriplegic who had vowed to kill himself if Brockman refused to operate on him.

Billy's parents were small people who resembled each other. They looked to be tough and hardworking, but their eyes were bright with fear now and they were timid before the Boss, as if in need of his approval.

"We didn't hurt him," Brockman began. "I know that for sure. How much we helped him—that remains to be seen."

They waited for more, but there was really nothing else to say. The tumor had to go to pathology before they would know what grade it was and how fast it was likely to return, and only time would tell about Billy's immediate recovery from the operation. Anything else he said would be psychology, not neurosurgery. Mind, if you like, not brain. Whatever it was, it wouldn't be delicate, or easy to take.

"The tumor was gelatinous. Like Jell-O, you know? Tapi-oca. I took it out with little copper spoons. Altogether"—he laid a finger across his thumb, just below the nail—"I'd say it was about this big."

When he said "Jell-O," Mrs. Eggleston flinched, and when he said "tapioca," she leaned against her husband. She was just beginning to straighten up when he pointed to his thumb, and then she almost collapsed.

Like a lot of big-name physicians, Brockman was known for his way with patients and families, but from the out-side it was sometimes impossible to comprehend his repu-tation. There were times when he waded through imposs-ible territory with grace, others—like this—when he was tactless, even cruel. What was remarkable, though, was that it didn't seem to matter to the people he addressed. So enormous was their need to believe in him that they ad-justed to what he said, rationalizing it so quickly that they looked to themselves for the source of their anxiety. If anything, they seemed to appreciate him most when he was at his roughest. As George Tinker explained, "Some-times he was brutal, but it never bothered me half as much as other doctors when they treated me like a baby. His honesty sort of made me honest with myself."

Brockman himself saw these meetings—like everything else in neurosurgery—as measures of courage. "Some surgeons will tell a patient, 'This may kill you, make you blind,' even though it isn't true. They're protecting their own asses. And others, they're so afraid of hurting the patient that they'll communicate their anxiety and make him even more frightened than he was when he came in. The truth is, every patient I see is scared to death, and there's nothing I can do about it. There's no certainty once you open somebody's head, and if you try to pretend there is, you won't fool him, only lose his confidence."

Other surgeons had different styles. Some were sweet and some funny, some maternal and ingratiating, some frigid, hard-nosed, and sadistic. One or two, the worst I saw, were seductive and childlike, trying to distract patients from their self-pity by being pitiable themselves. Altogether, Brockman's style struck me as adequate, no better or worse than anyone else's. Much has been written lately about the inability or unwillingness of most physicians to assist patients or families in their confrontations with death, but if—as Brockman noted often—the role of the surgeon is intervention, he would seem to be disqualified from the dialogue that such confrontations require. Brutal though it could be, Brockman's style seemed to be an acknowledgment of his proper role, an implicit bow to the truth: "I'll take care of the anatomy, and we'll leave the rest for your priest or your friends, or your boy when you meet again in the I.C.U."

The Egglestons had remained silent during his discourse, but now, as he prepared to leave, they came to life, firing all the questions they'd been harboring since Billy's symptoms had appeared. Was his speech endangered? His memory? Would he walk? Would he ever be able to swim? What about seizures? How much medication would he require? What should they tell his little sister?

Brockman dealt with them patiently, but he cut them off when he saw they meant to continue as long as he would let them. "Listen, we won't know about his tumor until the pathologists get to it. That will take a couple of days, then we'll talk again." He pointed to the copper bracelet Mrs. Eggleston wore. "Hey," he said, "that help your arthritis?"

"No." She laughed. "Not a bit."

"Too bad, huh? I tried one for a while and it didn't help me either. Okay, listen, I gotta go now. Billy should be in the I.C.U. by three this afternoon. You can see him as soon as he comes up."

He turned to leave, but still they held on, just as Duane Kirschner had held on that morning.

"He was happy-go-lucky!" cried Mr. Eggleston. "An athlete. He loved to run! He loved to swim! God, you should have seen—"

"Well, don't speak in the past," Brockman said. "He may be able to do it again. If that tumor doesn't come back, he'll be like any other kid his age."

But it seemed as if they had not heard him.

"Out of nowhere," said Mrs. Eggleston, "he gets this headache. Wakes up screaming in the middle of the night. 'I want to see a doctor!' he says. Can you imagine a kid wanting to see a doctor?"

Brockman backed off toward the elevator. "All right, then. I'll see you tonight when I make rounds. Why don't you have some lunch? The cafeteria's pretty good here, you know? Give yourselves a break, okay? Try to relax until you see him."

Although pediatrics was only two flights down, we had to take the elevator. Stairs were always locked here, protection against theft (especially of linen) that had lately been epidemic. It was a terrible inconvenience, a frequent subject at medical board meetings, but alternatives had yet to be found. What it meant, among other things, was that a doctor called to another floor on emergency was at the mercy of the elevators. And since elevator traffic was heavy all day, he could wait for ten or fifteen minutes while his patient waited one floor below.

The pediatric I.C.U.—where Brockman went now to see José's patient—was in the middle of the hall, halfway down the corridor near the nurses' station. Getting there was not a lot of fun. Ask any physician which specialty was the most depressing of his internship, and all except pediatric neurosurgeons will tell you: pediatric neurosurgery.

All the pain on any ward was unjust and incomprehensible, but here it could seem vicious. Along the way to the I.C.U. we passed an infant with a deformed face, two children in wheelchairs, another walking with a nurse's help, her head bandaged after craniotomy. There was a recreation room where a spastic child played billiards while rock music blasted from a jukebox. Pediatric neurosurgeons were the only ones I met who routinely explored what Brockman was exploring through me—involvement with patients *before* surgery, operation on a brain to which one was linked emotionally. In pediatrics it was possible to see a child reach up from her bed to embrace a surgeon, and watch him almost embarrassed as he let himself be hugged. Kenneth Beck gave the parents of his patients his home telephone number. "If you don't get depressed here," he told his residents, "you've got no business here." Pediatrics was different from adult neurosurgery because the risks were more easily justified, and the results were often unequivocal. It wasn't just a few more years you sought. You could turn a child around and send him off for a normal run, rebuild a face deformed at birth, cure hydrocephalus—which used to kill or cause extensive brain damage—with easily installed drainage tubes called shunts that drained fluid from the brain and disgorged it harmlessly in the belly or the heart (yes, the heart).*

The most distinctive thing about pediatrics was that it justified more aggression than adult surgery. When a full life span was at stake, there was a rationale for certain procedures that could not be justified with older patients. With the risks, however, the dangers increased as well. Surgery near the brain stem, such as the Boss had performed on Billy, would not often be risked on an adult, certainly not on an elderly person. But these regions, as

* Shunts had been around since 1957, and the technology was now so advanced that Beck could install one in fifteen minutes. Thanks to the CAT-scan, which permitted easy surveillance of their function, they could now remain in place for life (though sometimes the tubes had to be replaced). Beck at this time was following more than three hundred children with shunts he had installed.

noted, are volatile; occasionally a child would come through the surgery fine but never wake up or, like the child we saw before us now, bleed and go berserk with fever and convulsions.

She was eleven years old, thin as a reed and white as the sheet she lay on. Uncovered, naked on the bed (top sheets and pajamas obstruct the constant attention required by patients in the I.C.U.), her tongue protruded at the corner of her mouth and her fingers curled in half fists next to the guardrails. According to the tag on her wrist her name was Mary Ellen Bench. It wasn't a tumor that had brought her here but an arterial malformation (AVM in the vernacular), a deformity in one of the blood vessels which, like an aneurysm, can bleed and destroy surrounding tissue. The history was familiar: headaches, dizziness, inability to concentrate at school, suspicion that her problems were psychological, trips to a psychiatrist, consultation with the principal at school, and finally a grand mal seizure. She had entered the hospital two weeks ago and been kept under sedation for ten days. When her condition stabilized, Beck and José had operated on her successfully. Last night, as José had described, she had suddenly regressed, developed a fever of 105 degrees, and gone into convulsions. They had taken her back to the O.R. to see, first, whether she was hemorrhaging (she was) and, second, whether a shunt would relieve the symptoms (it did).

She had a tube in her mouth, an I.V. for nourishment in her left wrist, four electric sensors on her chest to track her EKG, an arterial line in the top of her right hand and another (for transfusions) in her foot, a blood-pressure cuff on her arm, a catheter in her urethra, an oxygen mask over her nose. Her skull was heavily taped, and the oscilloscope over her bed showed her blood pressure to be 90 over 70, which is very low indeed. They were keeping it down with a drug called furosemide, giving her steroids, mannitol, phenobarbital, and antibiotics through the I.V. Her eyes diverged, the way they sometimes do after surgery near the brain stem. Though her left eye stared at us, as we drew near, it was not possible to know if she was conscious. Behind her, on the railing, someone had draped one of those signs that decorate game rooms, offices, or luncheonettes where a touch of cuteness is desired. "Be nice to me," it said. "I've had a rough day."

As in the recovery room and the adult I.C.U. upstairs, the radio was a constant shriek—in a room, remember, where the lights were never turned out, where patients were drugged, confused, itching, prodded and turned and probed constantly, pained and terrified of pain to come and beginning, if conscious, to perceive the insult they'd experienced.

Brockman took hold of Mary Ellen's wrist and leaned close to her. "Hi, honey! How you feeling? I'm Dr. Brockman!"

She moaned softly, then rolled her head toward him on the pillow. Her left eye was fixed on him but her right gazed over his shoulder at the ceiling.

He turned to José. "How much mannitol?"

"Point-two-five grams per kilo," José said.

"Steroids?"

"One twenty-five every six hours."

"Anticonvulsants?"

"Phenobarb—thirty every six. No Dilantin yet."

Brockman let go of her wrist and fingered the unlit cigarette in his mouth (no smoking in the I.C.U.). "Nothing to do but wait. We can't give her any more. When she stabilizes get another scan. My hunch is she'll be okay by tomorrow evening. What's yours?"

"The same."

"Okay. Anything else you want me to see?"

José looked around the room. "Not really. We've got a meningo-myelocele over there and the kid with the aneurysm, both doing fine. What I'd really like you to see is the cranial-facial we did yesterday, but she's down in plastic surgery."

"Maybe tonight, after rounds."

"Okay. I'll check it out."

It was twelve thirty now, and we set off to find some lunch. At the elevator Brockman lit his cigarette and railed a bit at medical politics.

"You know what it costs to take care of that girl? A minimum of a thousand dollars a day, maximum of three. By the time she leaves here we'll have spent ten to fifteen thousand dollars on her,* but if she's a charity patient, the state will give us two hundred dollars a day. Not a penny more. They don't give a shit what disease we treat, it's still two hundred dollars a day. Do you know how much we could make if we filled this place with hernias?"

In the elevator he met the husband of a patient who was on the ward and a former patient, a gray-haired woman who was back at the hospital for outpatient radiation ("Come here," she cried, "and lemme kiss you!"), and on the ground floor we met Sarah Pincus, coordinator of the spinal-cord study, here to interview the husband of the woman who had thrown herself in front of a bus. She gave Brockman a quick summary of the patient's condition and then, as they parted, a nurse tapped him on the shoulder.

"Boss, can I speak to you a minute?"

"Later, Chris," he said. "After rounds."

On the street he lit another cigarette and waved his hand as if at mosquitoes. "I feel like I'm forty-seven tits and somebody sucking at every one. What were we talking about?"

We stopped at a coffee shop for sandwiches and coffee

---

* Hospital authorities estimate the cost for such a patient at $200 a day for a bed; $150 for every thirty minutes in the operating room; $500 to $1,000 for an angiogram; $150 for a CAT-scan; $3,500 for the surgeon's fee; $25 to $50 a day for medication; and $100 for any consultant who had to be called in.

and took them upstairs to his office. There were more than a dozen calls waiting for him, but all except two he stored with his secretary, for disposition later in the day. (When he had both the inclination and the time, he would send word to her office, and she would line up his calls, dialing the numbers two or three ahead, so he could proceed without interruption.) The first one he took now was from his friend in Washington, concerning the head-trauma grant —"Lemme fill you in, Bernie. They loved the clinical stuff. Ate up the stuff about blood flow"—and the second was from the aforementioned union leader, who he hoped would mediate the problem between the staff and the corporation. (Brockman: "War's gonna start any minute." Union Man: "Let it. After it's over, I'll come in and pick up the pieces.")

Besides a stuffed sand shark on the wall, the office was decorated with diplomas and citations and, of course, photographs: his father and grandfather, his teachers, and John F. Kennedy, who had been a personal friend. There was a green leather couch, a lovely Oriental rug on the linoleum floor, a desk lamp made out of an antique microscope. Simple as it was, I always thought of the room as a power center, an energy source, one of the few places I'd ever known from which authority proceeded without inhibition, apology, or doubt.

Brockman had been at Osler Memorial for eighteen years. Before that, beginning when he came out of the army at the age of twenty-eight, he had spent seventeen years at one of the prestigious hospitals on the West Coast. He had trained under two great neurosurgeons who had themselves trained with Harvey Cushing, and he had paid all the dues a neurosurgeon was expected to pay. At forty, he was perfectly accomplished as a clinician and a surgeon, but during the course of his training he had accumulated an ambition so large and diverse that anything short of a chairmanship seemed to him a dead-end street.

Since he had done pioneer work with tumors and pediatric neurosurgery and—spectacularly—angiography, his reputation, by this time, was already international. Offers of chairmanships began to pour in, and when he was forty-five he was offered what he wanted at Osler: a weak neurosurgical department in the midst of a fine medical school, a poor neurology department which he could shape according to his bias,* extensive clinical facilities, an endless supply of patients, money to expand in all directions.

When he came to Osler Memorial, there was no Intensive Care Unit in the entire hospital. There were three neurosurgical residents who got no supervision. There was no research under way, the anesthesia technique was horrendous, and the neurosurgical mortality statistics bordered on the criminal (though not available in the hospital's files, they were said to have been about 45 percent). The first time Brockman operated, he met the patient's parents as he went to the O.R. Having been told by the nurses that neurosurgical patients rarely left the hospital alive, they were on their way to pack their daughter's clothes and take them home. Brockman convinced them to hang around awhile. (The patient was cured and still comes in for annual examinations.)

Several weeks later, he and his staff expropriated a room, painted it themselves, attached blood-pressure machines to the walls, and called it an I.C.U. Within a year he had reorganized the process of resident selection and supervision, begun research into hydrocephalus, joined a

---

* Not long before, he had been offered another job at an equally famous hospital, but there the neurology department was headed by a man who was world-famous in his own right and as biased against surgery as Brockman was biased for it. After one meeting, the two had agreed that no institution was large enough for both of them. There were legendary tales about their battles over the years, but in fact they admired each other, and Brockman in particular spoke of his adversary with fondness.

large project in stroke research, and sent in his first application for federal money, a grant for aneurysm research that was rejected. Most important, he had cleaned up the surgical facility. Within five years, the technique at the hospital was as good as any in the world, already near its present 1 percent mortality rate, and within ten years it was on the map, one of the prominent neurosurgical departments in the world, famous especially for its work with aneurysms and for the teaching techniques that Brockman had pioneered.

Considering his position and his schedule, his desk was surprisingly neat, primarily because his letters and files were processed so quickly by his secretaries. Like many who've accumulated so much responsibility, Brockman (—as I've noted—) was absolutely dependent on his staff. There was a secretary who did nothing but type, and another who did nothing but insurance forms. The receptionist handled the phones, protecting him on that flank; another secretary was more or less in charge of residents and the applications (about one hundred a year) that came in for new positions; and a woman named Joan Buchanan directed the brain-tumor program as Sarah Pincus directed the spinal-cord project.

His principal guardians, however, were Claire Zerilla and Patricia Peterson. Both had been with him for more than fifteen years, and both lived in his apartment building, opposite the hospital, where he felt free to call on them at any hour of the day or night (for years they'd both been threatening to move, but neither had done anything about it). Pat was his clinical secretary—appointments, billing, follow-ups—and Claire was both department coordinator and nursemaid, responsible on the one hand for the day-to-day administration of departmental affairs, on the other for such personal matters as his checkbook. She typed and edited his papers, decided which charities he'd support and

how much he'd give to them, sent out his Christmas cards.
When he and his wife gave a party, she arranged the
catering and sent out the invitations. She ordered his
schedule (sometimes messing up; it was she who'd sent
him early to Denver), edited his papers, accepted or rejected his teaching appointments and invitations to lecture,
and generally made sure that he got where he was supposed to get with reasonable nods in the direction of punctuality. This last was no small part of her job, considering
that he served on thirty-seven different committees that
had to do not only with the medical center but also with
city, state, and federal affairs: he was chairman, for example, of the CAT-scan Committee within the city's Health
and Hospitals Corporation, a member of the Stroke and
Trauma Committee at the N.I.H., and a founding member
of the Pain Group, which was trying to build a center
where chronic pain would be investigated and treated as
an independent symptom.

At this time, Brockman owed Claire twelve weeks' vacation, but he left the room as if insulted if she mentioned
going away. Sometimes she raged at him (there was
enough love and hate between them to fuel a couple of
marriages), but mostly she took his dependency for
granted. "I never met a neurosurgeon who wasn't a baby,
and he's just like the rest. None of these guys can do
anything for themselves. They can't make decisions, and
they can't tolerate frustration. Once he got mad and threw
his cigarette lighter out the window. 'Don't come back,' he
says, 'until you find it.' The other day, Harvey got mad at
someone on the telephone and threw his briefcase across
the room, missed me by a couple of inches. They're all
crazy. Egomaniacs. It's like the better they function in the
O.R., the worse they are in the outside world."

Done with the telephone, Brockman turned to his dictating machine, snapping the switch with his thumb and listening to his own voice: "Mrs. Wesley has a walking prob-

lem, period. She's severely agitated and she manipulates her family, period. If we send her home, comma, she'll simply retire to enjoy her illness, period. New paragraph. Hopefully, if we keep her here . . ." He ran the machine forward, then stopped it again: ". . . can be of any further assistance, please don't hesitate to call, period. Uh—sincerely."

The phone beside him buzzed. "Yeah," he said, picking it up. "I'll talk to her." And then: "Hi, honey, how you doing? Still a lot of pain? Well, I think we better get you in here and let Dr. Ahmad examine you. What? Oh, no, I don't do backs any more. Dr. Ahmad is better than I am, one of the best in the world. Oh, no, no, I couldn't do that. I told you, I don't do backs any more. Listen, sweetie pie, everyone thinks I'm God, but I'm not, you know?"

He took up a file from a stack on his desk and leafed through it while he talked; then he buzzed Patricia, in her office next door, and had her arrange for the woman to see Ahmad. Two cigarettes simmered in the ashtray, smoking up the room, but now, dictating again, he lit another.

"Dr. Edmund Kress, Three Eastham Terrace, Hyannis, Massachusetts. Dear Dr. Kress.

"Just a note to describe surgery performed this morning on—uh—William Eggleston, the young man with left thalamic cystic tumor who you referred, period. Uh—this young man as you know was initially shunted for the relief of his—uh—increased intracranial pressure with good relief and at the time of his transfer to Osler Memorial Hospital he was intact from a neurological point of view, period. The only additional study was angiography which failed to show a very vascular blush which might have made me anxious about directly approaching this tumor, period. This was not seen and therefore through a posterior left midline approach the corpus callosum was split and the tumor cavity entered, period. Uh—the wall of the tumor was fairly firm and the center however was completely filled with gelatinous—uh—comma, grayish-pink material which could not be removed with suction but could be easily removed with—uh—small copper spoons. The tumor cavity was emptied and was spontaneously filling with fluid from the posterior portion of the left lateral ventricle at the completion of the procedure, period, new paragraph.

"When the pathological diagnosis is complete I will of course forward it to you. At this point I would expect it to be an astrocytoma of mild to moderate activity, comma, certainly not one which warrants chemotherapy, period. New paragraph.

"He will be maintained on phenobarbital—uh—thirty milligrams t.i.d. as a prophylactic anticonvulsant. I'll send you a report on his postoperative CAT-scan when we have it. Let us know if we can be of any further assistance and in the meantime—uh—comma, thanks for letting me help with this interesting problem. I of course would like to know how he does in the future. As always."

During the course of an average week, Brockman dictated sixty to eighty letters. When he traveled he took dictation equipment with him, and he was never without it at his country house on weekends. It may be that these days we all process encyclopedias like this, that anyone with large responsibility must be wired up to machines and secretaries, if only for protection from the flood. But he seemed uncomfortable unless overextended—an action junky who fortunately (for others as well as himself) found himself in the right place at the right time. The right talent for the right work and the opportunity to do it. The right century.

There was no limit on what he had to do, what others needed from him, what he needed from others, none on the extent to which he could communicate with other physicians or neural scientists (there were WATS lines in the office). The technology which made it possible to control intracranial pressure during surgery has also increased the opportunities for research and the means by which its results are disseminated and, with computers, the means by which it is stored and retrieved. But it was still Brockman who had to decide which journal to read, which footnote to pursue, which research to study, his brain which had to process the information and apply it. Where was the limit on what he had to know?

Journals and books simply flooded the office. For the small departmental library, there were subscriptions to twenty-two monthly journals and maybe half a dozen yearly symposia, but in the medical school library, downstairs, there were many more which could be called essential reading for neurosurgeons. Every specialty and subspecialty has several journals, and often the interdepartmental journals can be more valuable than the primary publications. A neurosurgeon is expected to keep himself abreast, among other fields, of pathology, angiography, CAT-scanning, neuropharmacology, neurochemistry, neurophysiology, neurobiology, trauma, epilepsy, hydrocephalus, electron microscopy, stroke, child neurology, psychiatry, anesthesia, immunology, vascular disease, cancer, meningioma, and spinal-cord damage. In 1977, more than half a million papers were published in the allied fields called the neural sciences, and no small number of those would expand into books. When I volunteered once to do work in speech pathology (another field a neurosurgeon might reasonably review), the therapist gave me what she called "an incomplete bibliography" to study before I began. It had nine hundred titles. As Lewis Thomas has written in an article published in *Science* magazine:

> The enterprise of biomedical research in the U.S. has expanded in scale and scope so greatly in the past thirty years that no one can begin to keep up with reading of it. It

used to be that a working immunologist could keep abreast of his field by covering three or four professional journals, plus *Nature* and *Science* for the first accounts of new observations. Now there are ten times that number of journals, each containing papers on immunology that cannot be overlooked, plus any number of monographs, review volumes, national and international symposium reports, and even a few newsletters. The journals are themselves five times their former size, with briefer articles and smaller print . . . so communication has become a serious problem, not only between scientists and the public, but among the scientists themselves.

As Thomas notes in the same article, one antidote to this impossible situation is gossip. More and more, scientists and physicians rely on their interpersonal contacts, gathering as much as they can from telephone conversations and incidental encounters (like breakfast in the cafeteria) and, most important, from national and international conferences. Brockman confessed to me once that he hardly read anything any more. "If I hear about something interesting, I get one of my boys to read it and tell me about it." As for conferences, there was seldom a time when he wasn't recently returned or about to go. Between this sort of trip and the others—equally important as far as his information file was concerned—when he went to teach or lecture, he made twenty to twenty-five trips in an average year, and a few of those were always international.

Nowadays we take the information explosion for granted,* but since we are concentrating on the organ of the body that processes our information and a surgeon

---

* Researchers at Bell Laboratories estimate that there is more information in a weekday edition of the *New York Times* than a person in the sixteenth century processed in a lifetime.

who processes that organ, it is worthwhile, I think, to
watch Brockman's wheels turn, check out the file drawers
that had to open and close in his mind, consider the neurons that had to fire, the shifts in time and identity and
language which had to take place for him to dictate these
letters, which later today would go out toward someone
else's desk and become another item in the information
flood.

> Dear Dr. Pasternak:
>
> I was distressed to see this attractive
> thirty-year-old housewife who as you know
> underwent lumbar laminectomy in September
> of 1976 by Dr. Peter Koburn for a right-sided
> L5-S1 lumbar disc.
>
> The history which she gave me prior to
> surgery was that of pain and numbness along
> the anterior aspect of both thighs, at times
> extending into her legs with a feeling of
> weight in her legs and paresthesia in both
> lower extremities. I reviewed her preoperative
> myelogram and she certainly did have a defect
> at the L5-S1 level on the right side; however,
> these symptoms are difficult to explain based
> on the myelographic deficit. Be that as it may,
> however, she has not made a very good
> recovery, as you well know.
>
> Her complaints now are pain in the coccyx
> and difficulty with sitting and walking, a
> sensation of "giving away" in the left leg and
> pains in both legs. I gather from the patient
> that Dr. Koburn has suggested now removal
> of the coccyx.
>
> It would be my opinion that further surgery
> would be seriously contraindicated in this
> young woman. In my experience, removal of
> the coccyx for coccygeal pain has really been

highly unsuccessful and I think that a second surgical procedure is pretty well doomed to failure in this young woman who has really not recovered from her first surgery. I have recommended to her as an alternative that she be referred to a formal program for her rehabilitation exercises for her low back and that she join a local health club for regular swimming and exercising in the water. I think she has to be handled quite firmly, indicating to her as I did that further surgery would only produce further deficit and that she must learn to work this out on her own with the help of rehabilitation therapy.

Dear Dr. Ashley:

I appreciate your information relative to the lack of adequate linen for the patients on the Surgical Service here at Osler Memorial. Clearly, the admission of private patients to Osler has served one of the purposes for which we had designed it; that is, to bring our attendings into closer contact with the patient population. Obviously the lack of clean linen is important for all our patients, including the private admissions, and I will be talking this problem over with administration. Thank you for your attention.

Dear Dr. Porter:

Just a note concerning Mrs. Mannes, who underwent mediastinoscopy followed immediately by thoracotomy and excision of her peripheral carcinoma of the lung.

She was protected during her operative period with the use of corticosteroids. She had some period of confusion and disorientation during her time spent in the I.C.U. This likely was somewhat related to the presence of her huge right frontal lobe tumor, but, of course, can be seen in patients in the I.C.U. without known intracranial disease.

Corticosteroids were rapidly tapered and she cleared entirely and has now been discharged from the hospital to be followed by Dr. Martinez from the point of view of her thoracic problem and by you in terms of her further neurological evaluation.

If she is "cured" of her chest tumor and if, after an appropriate period of follow-up, this seems to be definite, one probably ought to consider eventual removal of her meningioma.

As you would know, our eminent colleague, Ed Melik, was convinced that she would get into trouble in her postoperative period. We may have been skating on thin ice during her period of confusion but at times I guess it is better to be lucky than smart.

During the next half hour there were eight more letters. Two went to insurance companies to verify operations and assist patients in their claims; one to the State Motor Vehicle Bureau, to recommend a driver's license for a patient who had suffered from seizures (most states forbid such people to drive until they have had two years seizure-free); one to a tumor immunologist he was trying to hire in order to broaden his department and improve its chance for a large tumor grant that would soon be available through the N.I.H. One concerned a seventy-year-old lady who had been having seizures for twenty years and now, after surgery, was dying rapidly; one—copies to be sent to five different hospitals—recommended a former resident for "privileges" in neurosurgery; one described an epic of an iatrogenic tragedy, a fifty-five-year-old man who had had an unnecessary back operation two years before and was now in a state of constant, excruciating pain, a Demerol addict, suicidally depressed, with nothing in the least abnormal on any of his X-rays; and the last one, finally (a bit redundant because he was so embarrassed by her), concerned Rosie Galindez.

> I am distressed to have to write to you concerning Mrs. J. C. Galindez, who was seen in the office with clear evidence of displacement of her frontal flap and a disfiguring bony protuberance at the midline. This is obviously not a serious matter but it is distressing to Mrs. Galindez. I suggested that her flap be replaced with as small an incision as possible, sparing her nicely regenerating head of hair. It is not a serious matter but obviously both she and I were distressed by this complication.

Meanwhile, the telephone had not stopped. Most of the calls were held up by the receptionist, but those that came through were equal to the letters in the demands they made on him. He had a screaming argument with one caller, a touchy time with someone from the University of Florida who wanted him to lecture, a call from a friend who wanted to meet him for lunch, an emergency consultation with the mother of a boy who had fallen off a roof and now lay paralyzed in a suburban hospital. Benny had come in twice with angiograms to review, and Harvey had stopped by to report on his meeting with the Alfredo family (at this point they wanted surgery; tomorrow they wouldn't).

Now Claire sat down with Brockman to review his upcoming schedule.

"Number one, you're giving a paper Monday morning at eleven on subarachnoid hemorrhage."

He had taken out his appointment book, and he took notes as she spoke, like a student attending to a professor. "At the V.A.?"

"Right. And after that you've got the lunch meeting of the Emergency Medical Board. Better review the material on heroin because that's what they want to discuss."

The phone rang. "Yeah, yeah. I know. . . . Well, why not? Why the fuck not? Get on it. I don't care what they say. We've got to have it!" He slammed the phone down, lit a cigarette. "Where were we? Heroin? I know that stuff. No need to look at it. Go ahead."

"The next Saturday at nine thirty, there's a meeting of the Trauma Committee, and then Tuesday you go down to Washington for the N.I.H. presentations. The following Thursday, you're going to Jerusalem as visiting professor, and you'll give the brain-tumor course over that weekend. After that, you're back here until the Cushing Conference on May first in Toronto. You'll be there until the sixth, give your paper at the lunch meeting, leave that evening for San Francisco. You've got a day open there for fishing. Do you want me to reserve the boat?"

"No. I'll talk to them myself."

"May thirteenth is the N.I.H. Brain Tumor meeting. You'll come back here the same day, and May fourteenth and fifteenth you'll give the spinal-cord course here."

The phone rang again. "Yeah? Well, tell him I need to talk to him. Just tell him that, you understand? Tell him I need to talk to him!" He slammed the phone down. "Goddamn it, he's gotta stop that shit. What's after the spinal cord?"

"June looks good. We'll have the visiting neurosurgeons from Japan, but we got out of the Green Bay conference. Unless they wheedle you into the Florida thing, you'll have an easy month. June nineteenth is the aneurysm paper in Portland. Should I go into July?"

"No, no. Shit, I'm exhausted. Just make sure you send

a copy of the schedule to my wife so she'll believe me, okay?''

Claire removed a letter from her file. "Do you want to answer this?"

"What's it about?"

"You questioned something in the *Journal of Neurosurgery* last fall. This guy says you're wrong."

"Leave it. I'll have a look later."

He put out his cigarette and put another in his mouth, though—asserting himself against the habit—he wouldn't light it for another five minutes. Leaning back in his chair, he spread his feet on the desk until he looked like a pregnant woman about to deliver.

"What about the applications?"

"The spinal cord is ready, but not the brain tumor. They have to be in at the end of the month."

"Okay. Make a note for me to meet with Harvey on the tumor project. We've got to find an immunologist."

Claire stood up to go. "By the way," she said, "isn't it time you saw Betty Abraham?"

"Why should I see her?"

"Her mother says she's losing her memory."

"Bullshit. Her mother pesters her all day long. If there's anyone I ought to see, it's her."

After Claire left, he made a couple of telephone calls, then headed downstairs to the office in which he saw his private patients.

Patricia had been there for half an hour when he arrived, and the waiting room was full of patients, some of whom had waited months for their appointments. All of them— unless they were priests, nuns, rabbis, or policemen, all of whom he not only examined but operated on without charge—would pay $75 for their visit and, if they went to surgery, $2,000 for craniotomy. The figure was close to the national average but decidedly low for a man of his promi-

nence. Brockman paid little attention to his fees. According to Claire, he had bragged when he raised his craniotomy fee to $1,500, unaware that many of his colleagues,
at other hospitals, were charging twice as much. Now the
same disparity remained. Some charged as much as $5,000
for craniotomies. Even Kellogg and Beck charged more
than he did for some procedures.

The file drawer that opened now was called neurology.
He examined patients much as a neurologist would, checking for balance ("Close your eyes . . . hold out your hands
. . . touch your nose . . ."), auditory or visual distortion,
peripheral nerve damage, deciphering clues like a detec-
tive ("If a person walks without swinging his arms, it may
be due to rigidity or spasticity, but if you can't find evidence of this, you look for cerebellar disease on the same
side"), exploring distortions in perception that might have
captivated a philosopher. For example, did the shooting
pains in this first patient's legs derive from a herniated
disk, or a tumor in the spinal cord, or a lesion in the brain
which affected the nerves connecting to her thighs? Or was
it a neurochemical disturbance that made her hypersensitive to pain, or—conversely—did she lack those neurochemicals called endorphins, which suppress sensations of
pain? Or was her pain not physical but psychological (if
one could pretend this had nothing to do with the brain!),
arising, say, from certain problems that made her infantile
in the presence of pain, causing her to use it as a means
of seduction or control? Was her pain really excruciating
or was it imagined, and if it was imagined was there not
something about the alchemy of imagination that made it
real? Doesn't the imagination affect the brain at least as
much as the brain affects the imagination?

Since most of his patients were referred by neurologists,
there was seldom need for a thoroughgoing neurological
examination. The question now was whether to admit
them to the hospital for workup toward surgery or send

them back to their neurologists or internists for less radical treatment. It wasn't an easy decision, nor was it easy on the patients, but they were more often relaxed than frightened in his presence, and some seemed relieved to be there. As I've noted, they'd usually had their share of indecision, and there was a sense that, having gotten to the neurosurgeon, their voyage, for better or worse, would soon be over.

The second patient was James, a freaky fellow in his early twenties, tall, dark-haired, and gangly, laughing constantly at nothing in particular. Six months before, Brockman had removed a tumor of his acoustic nerve—a lesion which had caused severe hearing disorder—and James, who had a history of chronic schizophrenia as well as brain tumor, reported now that he knew he was well because he could talk to himself again.

After he left (and after the Boss had confirmed that he was in excellent shape), I asked what James had meant. Brockman shrugged. "The guy is crazy." So much, I thought, for the mind-brain distinction. The man who had looked into James's brain and even touched it was locating his mental problems elsewhere.

"Do you think his surgery or his tumor had anything to do with making him crazy?" I asked him.

"Frankly, no."

"Then the mind and brain are absolutely separate for you?"

"Not necessarily," he said. "Talking about the mind topographically is like talking about the end of space. It makes no sense at all. The only people who get away with it are senile neurosurgeons and neurologists at the end of their careers. They think they've got to sum it up, explain the whole of existence via the mitochondria or some such shit. God spare me that kind of ego trip."

The next patient was a handsome Puerto Rican woman in her late forties. She too had recovered from surgery (meningioma), but she was babying herself, staying in bed most of the day and living on welfare. "Most of your problem is in your head," he told her (as if the tumor he had removed had been somewhere else). "What you've got to do, Maria, is go back to work."

"Okay," she said. "The doctor say work, Maria go to work. When I come back to see you?"

"You don't have to make an appointment. Just call me up if anything goes wrong. If not, you don't have to see me."

"Can't I just come back to kiss you?"

A smile flickered, but he turned it off. "Watch it now, sweetie. You'll ruin my reputation."

She reached for his hand. "Oh, you're one lovely doctor. I sure happy to see you."

He stood up from his desk and went to the door. "Okay, honey. You be good now. Once you're back at work, you'll be amazed how good you feel."

On her way out, she gave it one more try, stopping face-to-face and staring into his eyes. "If you ask me, what I need is one good man."

"Maybe you do, maybe you do," Brockman said. "And when you find him, tell him your neurosurgeon says there's nothing in your brain to hold you back."

Two patients with back problems followed her, both referred to health clubs, and then there was a beautiful Jamaican woman with a pituitary tumor (confirmed by angiograms she brought from another hospital). Obviously it had to come out, but since she was a nurse and knew a bit about neuroanatomy and the location of the pituitary gland in the depths of the brain, she was especially frightened of surgery.

"How they gonna get to my pituitary gland without digging a hole in my brain?" What she didn't know was that she would benefit from the new technique of approaching the pituitary through the upper lip and gums.

This extremely difficult operation had become almost routine, but it was not an easy thing for the patient to deal with, especially if the one who described the procedure viewed it, as Brockman did, strictly as a surgeon.

"Nothing to worry about," he assured her happily. And spreading his lips like an actor in a toothpaste commercial, he pointed his finger at his upper gums. "We go right through your upper lip, then plug up your nose with a piece of cartilage."

Unless patients came alone, they were seldom addressed. Like many physicians and surgeons, Brockman had a tendency to talk of them in the third person—"This man's got to come in the hospital" or "There's no reason why she can't drive a car"—as if they were not quite present. Sometimes he did not look at them at all but spoke entirely to the family or friend who'd brought them in. Most of the older women (especially if postoperative) seemed to be slightly in love with him, and almost all the women related to him sexually. ("God, he's cute," said one to her husband, when Brockman left the room.) In general, while he made jokes, they seldom did, and even when he looked directly at them, their eyes were almost always downcast, as if he had brought out all their diffidence, as if, like the Egglestons, they needed not just his help but his sanction.

It was a clear-cut, stable relationship, a quintessential model, from a certain point of view, for all dependencies, and since all the need was on one side and all the power on the other, its magical quotient was not insignificant. Unfortunately the dangers of the magic, as Eric J. Cassell has written in *The Healer's Art*, were not insignificant either:

> It is interesting that perhaps the seemingly most omnipotent of all physicians are the neurosurgeons, and theirs is the specialty in

which nature's odds are most against them. In
terms of curing, they are the least effective.
In addition, they operate on the brain, the
most mysterious part of the body. Does any
diagnosis strike such terror as a brain tumor?
The brain surgeon's incredible feeling of
omnipotence helps protect us from our fear.

The same sense of omnipotence that
protects the patient endangers the doctor
because he is rarely aware of it or its place in
medical care. Omnipotence is magical power; it
defies the realities of life. As time goes on the
distinctions between magic and reality become
hazy and the magic is reinforced—reflected in
the patient's eyes. Error may become, in the
doctor's mind, less possible, and he stands the
danger of functioning primarily with magic
rather than with knowledge. He heals . . . but
may begin to fail in curing as his knowledge
lags. Once he begins to believe that he, rather
than his knowledge and technical skill, is the
source of the cure, danger lurks in the image
reflected back from his patient's eyes. If the
doctor looks into those eyes, the image that he
sees is—God. But that image is the enemy.

Pause then to consider the situation from Brockman's
point of view, the difficulty of keeping things in some kind
of rational perspective. Gazed at with reverence day after
day, feeding on that reverence, lifted by it on bad days,
manic from it if you started off high, distracted by it from
self-doubt, personal problems, or fear of death—what
more did you need on days when you didn't know why you
were alive than to look in their eyes and believe what you
saw? Think how difficult it must be to keep on learning and
criticizing yourself, and to deal with the awareness that
your skill and intelligence, however great they might be-

come, would always be dwarfed by the astonishing mystery you faced. Early on he must have learned to use anxiety, transform it into energy that turned his patients on, but as Cassell notes, the power and adulation that seemed to be his great reward could keep him out of the lab, make him lazy about his reading (or his attention to the residents who read for him; had it made him lazy already?), satisfy him with 40-percent removal of a tumor when he might have got 75. More seriously, it could destroy the innocence which, as any good physician will tell you, is the prerequisite for good medical practice, which alone permits the fresh perception of a patient that each new case requires. The plain fact of it was that neurosurgery bred arrogance and humility at equal rate, power over death and constant awareness of it, a conjoined belief in human dignity and human futility which had so long been part of Brockman's day that it no longer seemed like a paradox. When patients looked at you as if you were God, and what you most desired was to believe them, it wasn't easy to remember your ignorance, but that—exactly—was what you had to do.

7

A Bounty of Mementos

For an outsider, the hospital was an endless succession of mind trips, a kind of recapitulation of all the different strategies one's mind had evolved for dealing with or denying what it could not comprehend. All days were voyages, some marked with insight, even catharsis, others almost deadening in their monotony. The worst were those when everything you saw—suffering, courage, bewilderment (in staff as well as patients), or comedy—was trivialized, food for gossip, isolated images one collected like a tourist. Hanging around with surgeons, it was easy for that to happen. Pain was filtered through their authority, disasters became "cases," and patients were mediums through which one affirmed one's excellence and compassion. It wasn't as if the doctors didn't care—far from it—but what lifts the spirits like pain one can alleviate? The great danger was that if you became, as you must, addicted to this reversal, you were blinded to the truth of what was going on around you. And if you were blinded to this truth, you could forget about the others. If brain damage didn't touch you, nothing would.

But fortunately the addiction was imperfect. On days

when it failed, it was as if you'd come out of anesthesia. Leaning half asleep against the wall in the operating room, you'd tune in suddenly to what was happening, and it would scare you to death or—amazingly enough—exhilarate you, strip you of your self-importance and sometimes your identity as well. Human beings, after all, were dismantled here, relieved first of consciousness, then piece by piece of their organic singularity. Like those patients Brockman wanted to hibernate at minimum EEG, they lived for a time on the peripheries of the void, the edge where material became and ceased to be animate, where life and death were so near to indistinguishable that they could seem synonymous (was it joy or terror that came with this perception?). And those who observed such patients in their travels, who came to the hospital with everyday pride and identity, minds filled with the usual descriptions and discriminations, could be dismantled emotionally and intellectually as the patients were dismantled physically. Indeed, observers could take a trip that paralleled the patients', with one enormous difference—remaining conscious, they perceived the void that was negotiated. Unlike the patients, they'd remember what happened here, and that memory could never in any fundamental sense be assimilated. How could it? It was a recollection of nonexistence which the very act of memory denied.

How one drank at this particular well was dependent on one's own capacity and availability. Many days, when things were trivial, I did not drink at all. Everything was television, hopelessly remote. Looking over the Boss's shoulder, I would think, That's a human brain! and there was no connection between the thought, the object it described, and the mind to which the thought was addressed. But often, when the anesthesia began to fail, my mind was fixated and desperate, everywhere but in the room. It wasn't normal distraction but something more, neurological rather than psychological, it seemed to me, as if my brain were having a temper tantrum or, more exactly, a seizure. Often, too, the distraction became self-consciousness, a descent into extremities of reflection which are not, from what I hear, uncommon to those who explore the neural sciences. I would see the patient's brain as my own, imagine my own mentation occurring in that flesh, my thoughts a chemical, synaptic process, *this* view of *that* brain pulsating along *my* optic nerve. Such moments could become almost mystical, as if by recognizing the materiality of thought, you had driven a wedge between your own thought process and your identity. They could also be ridiculous, parodies of intellectualism, as if you were trying simultaneously to embrace materialism and think your way around it, the secret thought an oxymoron: If I know I'm just material, then I've got to be more! In retrospect, such excursions often seemed like rides on a merry-go-round in a hall of mirrors, one more joke among many that neurosurgery contrived.

On those rare days when distraction ceased and the mind focused, the silence was riveting, but the emotions that grew from it were no less ambivalent than anything else about the hospital. Sometimes I found it all a kind of liberation, as if the absurdity and hopelessness had forced me to relinquish everything, give up the dreams and attachments which over the years had become my principal sources of despair. Other days I held on tight, like a drowning man clinging to a raft. There was no way to predict which way I'd go, but for this very reason the operating room and the ward became perfect, often painful, mirrors, offering clear and irrefutable pictures of where I was at any particular moment on a given day.

Once the mirror showed a spectacular B movie, a comedy in retrospect, that scared me to death when it happened. Brockman did a hemispherectomy that morning, removing half the brain of a twenty-two-year-old man named Marvin Welsh. Standing at his shoulder, maybe twelve inches from the brain he'd just exposed, I flashed that I would push his hand, drive it with his scalpel into Marvin Welsh's flesh. It was nothing but a flash at first, just another suicidal impulse, like the urge to jump from skyscrapers or put your finger in an electric fan. Images gathered—blood spurting, screams, panic—but I entertained them with detachment. Just a few neurons, I told myself, misbehaving in my brain. I saw it all as an amusement, a freak show that happened to be subjective. But gradually the impulse deepened and spread. First it seemed possible, then probable, and then all at once—no more laughter now—absolutely certain. Eventually I became so frightened that I actually retreated to a corner of the room and stood with my arms crossed, as if protecting them from themselves, until the attack was over.

I had never felt anything like that before, and I never did again, but it seemed to me a perfect summation of the conflict that neurosurgery could engender in the mind. Whatever path you took as you wound your way through the labyrinth, there was one element you'd never escape: awareness of the brain and your helplessness before it. No matter how you might trivialize or rationalize the experience, there was no way around the realization, conscious or unconscious, that you were absolutely dependent on this ridiculous piece of flesh. That without its help you could not breathe or see or hear or talk or make love or tie your shoe or remember your name. That the death or dysfunction of a few errant cells could paralyze you, make you mute, cause an epileptic fit, or, as my brain had just informed me, release violence sufficient to take a man's life.

Seizures like this, while observing neurosurgery, were finally the reactions of the mind to this bit of news about the brain, the mind attempting to comprehend that which, by definition, was beyond comprehension. If language and memory are dependent on the brain, then so is thought, so is comprehension, so is the mind itself, and how do you think about that? How does the mind comprehend its own materiality, when comprehension is itself an attempt to transcend the limitations of matter?

The circularity was endless when these questions arose. They were crystallizations of the mind-brain argument which has teased philosophers and scientists and theologians for centuries. For sure, you did not answer the questions, but you understood, I believe, at certain moments, why they could not be answered: the hopelessness of an investigation in which the goal was identical with the means by which one sought to achieve it. Whether or not the understanding made a difference—that's another story. Mostly, I think, it was processed as you had processed understandings all your life—remarked and stored, recollected and forgotten, distorted, exaggerated, deepened, and eviscerated. The circularity, in other words, continued. You could as easily remember the end of your memory or imagine your own death as think about the limitations of your thought. And the distraction and violence, the B movies and—on another level—the sexuality that Brockman had remarked, were nothing more, it seems to me, than strategies for dealing with the frustration, the absurd comedy that the brain poses when you meet it, as the surgeons liked to say, in the flesh.

The justification for Marvin Welsh's operation was his seizures, which, having resisted all other forms of treatment, had increased in frequency during the past two years until they now occurred every four or five minutes. He had been retarded and hemiplegic, his right hemisphere dysfunctional, since an attack of encephalitis when he was nine months old, and the hope was that the hemispherectomy, which would excise his dead hemisphere, would cure his seizures without further damaging his brain. Though hardly routine, the operation was not so difficult. There are no hidden arteries to worry about when an entire hemisphere is removed, no crucial functions to protect. Brockman simply chopped it apart as if making it into a jigsaw puzzle. The crowd that morning in the O.R. was due less to the exotic nature of the procedure (they rarely did this sort of thing any more) than the opportunity it offered for review of one's neuroanatomy. How often except on cadavers did one get to see the anterior aspect of the cerebellum (not removed) or the midline of the left temporal lobe?

When dissection was complete, the Boss sent for Beck, who had just completed an operation down the hall, and reconstructed the excised hemisphere for him. It was in three large pieces, in paper cups on the instrument table, and piece by piece, as if trying out the puzzle, he restored it to the cavity and took it apart again.

"Do you see, Ken? First you do a frontal lobectomy. Amputate the thalamus here, then come down here, across the temporal lobe, following this line. From there on, it's just a matter of logic."

Since I had forgotten by this time that Marvin was alive (though one could discern a pulse in veins at the bottom of the cavity), it came as a surprise to hear the Boss interject, in the midst of this demonstration, "What's the pressure? Okay. Don't let it go higher. He's starting to ooze from all over. I don't want any blood in this cavity when we close it."

He did not fill the cavity with Ping-Pong balls, as old-timers are said to have done. Instead, since they had learned by now that the brain would produce sufficient cerebrospinal fluid to fill itself, he spread oxidized cotton (which would be absorbed) along its surface and closed the dura loosely. He had opened the dura at nine fifteen and he closed it at eleven forty-five, accomplishing a procedure in two and a half hours which, according to Beck, would have taken most any other surgeon six or seven. (The opening of the skull had taken an additional hour, and the closing would add another hour.) When he was done, he hurried to the locker room, dressed quickly, grabbed a taxi for the airport, flew down to Washington for an N.I.H. meeting, and returned at four thirty, to check out Marvin in the I.C.U.

I had lunch in the locker room with Harvey Kellogg, who had an aneurysm scheduled next in the room where Marvin Welsh was being closed, and Ken Beck, who had another patient on the way down. It was not unusual for either of them to do more than one procedure in a day. Just the week before, Ken had done three in one morning, the patients' weight—combined—nine and a half pounds. Those were shunts, a procedure which had become more or less routine. This morning, most definitely, had not been routine. Working with José, Ken had excised an arterial malformation (AVM) almost identical to the one he had removed for Mary Ellen Bench, the little girl I'd seen with Brockman in the I.C.U.

Now, while Harvey and I waited, Ken sat down behind us at the telephone to dictate his notes on the operation.

> Under satisfactory general endotracheal anesthesia with central and arterial pressure monitoring, the patient was placed on the O.R. table in the supine position with the head turned toward the left side. A large hemicraniectomy-type of scalp flap was outlined, the anterior limb of which took its origin above the bridge of the nose, and the posterior limb of which terminated well behind the right ear.

Speaking as if reading, without hesitation or inflection, he sounded exactly like one of the first brain-damaged patients I had met, a man named Sam Cramer, who had stroke damage on the right side of his brain. Sam had

retained language as—according to brain localization theory—he was supposed to have done, but his speech was
devoid of music or rhythm or any variation of tone. It is
only one of the difficulties of such theory that while "language" is generally located on the left side and "musical
aptitude" on the right, the interdependence of these two
functions is generally ignored. Like Ken's voice now,
Sam's might have been automated. Even more remarkable, they resembled each other, at this moment, in point
of view as well as intonation. Like many brain-damaged
people, Sam's mind was specific and concrete, lacking in
abstraction and imagination. He had his language and his
reason, but he lacked its normal extensions into meaning
and generalization. Ask him how he felt and he would talk
about his arm or his leg, speak of himself as if he were an
object. Ask if he were happy or sad, and he would look at
you without comprehension. Though he could carry on a
perfectly adequate conversation, speaking with him could
be as difficult and disconcerting as speaking with Raymond Dreyer—even more so, because Sam seemed to be
all right. It was impossible to say what was missing in his
speech.

Ken's speech at this moment was not terribly different from Sam's; it was focused, concrete, external, void
of emotion, indifferent to the implications of what it described. Almost as though his work and the recollection
of it now engaged one region of his brain to an extent
that suppressed the others, strengthened that part
which related to the external world objectively, and
weakened those others which might have surrounded
his memory with emotion, broken down his separation
from what he observed, extended it in time with meaning and implication. It was as though his world, at this
moment, had three dimensions, not four. His mind was
essentially that of the technician Brockman had described: a manipulator of objects, an interventionist, a

manager of power. Pejorative though this description
sounds, the state of his mind was, in fact, a measure of
his competence and concentration. He was exactly what
his work required him to be. One had only to listen to
him, see how he had spent his morning, to realize that
he could not be anything else.

> The incision was carried down to the bone,
> and hemostasis was obtained with Raney clips.
> Then, utilizing periosteal elevators, a
> full-thickness scalp flap was reflected including
> pericranium. Following this, the coronal and
> sagittal sutures were identified, and burr holes
> were placed for the bone flap, one inch off the
> midline, and inferiorly in the region of the
> temporal bone.

After a complex description of the bone flap and the
subsequent dissection of the brain beneath it, he detailed
how they had arrived "approximately one and one half
centimeters beneath the cortical surface" at the malformation. The challenge at this point became one of orientation,
as various landmarks, visible within the brain, were
related to those that weren't, so that dissection would not
endanger arteries or vital function.

> The falx was identified . . . brain was then
> retracted from it . . . and the free surface of
> the falx as well as the opposite cingulate
> gyrus was visualized. The corpus callosum
> was ultimately visualized, and then the
> enormous feeding anterior cerebral artery
> from the right side was identified.

Piece by piece, the vessels that fed the malformation
were identified, coagulated, and cut. "It was of interest,"
he noted, "that the extreme turbulence which had been

noticed in the aneurysm* ceased after ligation of the temporal feeders. An attempt was made to spare what was
interpreted to be the precentral gyrus" (i.e., because it
controlled language function).

> In the posterior inferior region of the
> cortical resection a large clot was encountered,
> and this was suctioned out. Utilizing blunt
> dissection, the aneurysms, which numbered
> about three and were approximately the size
> of a lemon, were gradually mobilized from the
> interior of the brain. Finally, the venous
> aneurysms and the remainder of the feeders
> were rolled out, and a number-zero silk suture
> was placed around the pedicle medially,
> following which the entire malformation was
> removed in one piece.
> Hemostasis was obtained. The pressure
> which had been maintained at hypotensive
> levels was permitted to return to normal, and
> again hemostasis was obtained. Oxidized
> cotton was placed around the margins of the
> brain removal. A number-sixteen French
> catheter was placed at the site of the brain
> removal to serve as a drain, following which
> the dura was closed with interrupted four-oh
> silk sutures. The bone flap was replaced after
> obtaining hemostasis again, and bone chips
> were placed in the burr holes. The patient
> returned to the recovery room in satisfactory
> condition.

When Ken was done, he resumed normal speech with
only the slightest pause to get his bearings, and then he

---

* AVMs sometimes produce an aneurysm in an adjoining vein. What
Beck was probably referring to here, however, was a venous dilation
caused by the pressure from the AVM—not, strictly speaking, an aneurysm.

and Harvey and I bought sandwiches off the refreshment cart and took them back to the locker room. They were old friends, colleagues for twelve years now, and generally they laughed a lot when they were together, but this morning they were out of sorts, grumbling while they ate. As it happened, they were both at the tail end of a series of catastrophes and misadventures which had broken down, for both of them, the bemused detachment they liked to affect with regard to their work.

Though neither liked to review cases (both of them being, like Brockman, the sort of men who dropped things quickly when they were done), events had overwhelmed them this time, and when I inquired about the reasons for their anger, they answered with enthusiasm, as if competing to see whose mood was fouler, whose luck had been worse during the previous twenty-four hours. Their primary complaint was with Brockman, who yesterday morning had removed their clothes from the locker they shared and thrown them on the floor in the anesthesiologists' equipment room. Lately, it seemed, several anesthesiologists had been sneaking space in the locker that Brockman shared with Ken and Harvey, and yesterday, finding no room for his own clothes, Brockman had decided to teach them a lesson. Bundling all the clothes together, he had dragged everything down the hall to a room where no one would think to look for it, and Harvey and Ken, returning from their operations, had found themselves with no clothes but their scrub suits until nine in the evening, when they met the Boss and he admitted what he'd done. Brockman, as often, had charmed them out of their anger (no great problem, this, since neither had entirely overcome the fear of him they'd felt since beginning their residencies), but now, as they recounted their story and realized, I think, that they had forgiven him too easily, they lived it all over again.

As it happened, this had been the prelude for much worse things to come. The operation from which Harvey had returned, when he found his clothing gone, was an apparently successful pituitary tumor, but he was still waiting for his patient to wake up (she did, later that afternoon, and went home ten days later). And last evening, with her on his mind, and tickets for him and his son to a Rostropovich concert (they were both cellists, and Rostropovich was their hero), he had met—still dressed in his scrub suit—with the Alfredo family, having scheduled Victor's operation (with their approval) for this morning. Though the meeting was expected to be routine, a kind of review of all the information on anastomosis which they had heard several times before, Dominic had become anxious and argumentative, turned on Harvey, and accused him of malpractice because he hadn't removed the aneurysm two years before (when Harvey actually had wanted to remove it; Dominic had blocked him then as well). Finally, after drawing out the meeting until half an hour after the Rostropovich concert had begun, Dominic had decided that surgery was out of the question and insisted that Victor go home with them at once.*

Ken listened to Harvey patiently, but then he shook his head. "Harvey, if I'd had a day like that, I'd consider myself on vacation. Remember Mickey, that eight-year-old girl who came to us from the cancer clinic?"

"The astrocytoma?"

"Yeah, that's the one. We did her tumor, let's see, ten days ago, and she was doing great until yesterday morning. Suddenly gets this rash all over her body. Fever goes up to one hundred and seven. I called the clinic to see if they could explain it. 'Oh, yeah,' they say, 'she's anergic from chemotherapy.' Which means, of course, that she can't take blood transfusions unless the new blood is ir-

---

* Two weeks later, the same operation was performed on Victor by a surgeon in California, who then telephoned Harvey and asked him to follow up postoperatively. "Of course," Harvey said. "Tell the sonofabitch to call me up."

radiated. And since we happen to have given her six quarts during surgery, we've almost certainly lost her."

"Of course we have," Harvey said. "Why didn't they tell you she'd had chemotherapy?"

Ken shrugged. "Slipup, they said. They apologized, of course. Everyone makes mistakes, et cetera. While I was talking to her parents, she went into shock, secondary to massive bleeding. I had to leave the meeting to resuscitate her."

"What happens now?"

"We've sent her back to the clinic. The only hope, they say, is massive doses of chemotherapy."

"Of course. Obliterate the white cells and the bone marrow. If that works, I'd call it a miracle, wouldn't you?"

"Absolutely. I'd be surprised if she's alive this evening."

"Is that all?" Harvey said.

"Christ," said Ken. "I wish it were. Wait till you hear the rest."

After meeting with Mickey's parents, Ken had come down to the O.R. to do a shunt, returned to the locker room to find his clothes missing. The rest of the day was one disaster after another. Three families to see: one child inoperable, two to be done as soon as possible. The inoperable child was two days old, born with a birth defect called meningomyelocele which would make him a neurological and orthopedic disaster, and one of the operable kids was suffering from meningitis, a delayed effect from a previous operation for brain tumor six weeks before. During one of these meetings Ken was called on an emergency to the radiology department, where a patient undergoing embolization—ostensibly one of the safer neurosurgical procedures—had had a seizure and hemorrhaged on the table. By the time he reached her she was dead. An "intact" twenty-six-year-old woman who had been expected to leave the hospital in a week, she was Brockman's patient, and

since he was at a meeting, it fell to Ken to meet with
her family and break the news.

Harvey and I heard him out, sat with blank, dumb faces
for a moment, and then—at the same time—broke up
laughing. How else, except with tears, was such a tale to
be received? Even Harvey, iciest of all the staff, had to
admit that Ken had overstated the case for neurosurgical
melodrama. "Ken," he said, "the trouble with you is that
you've got no sense of proportion. Who would believe that
sort of day if they saw it on television?"

Beck and Kellogg were Brockman's principal disciples,
the men who would take over the department (unless outsiders were brought in) when he retired. Both in their early
forties, they came out of backgrounds similar to his, but
their differences were as interesting as their similarities.
All three shared medical backgrounds, doctor fathers who
could finance their seemingly endless educations, and all
had decided very early that medicine was what they
wanted to do. (Harvey knew he would be a neurosurgeon
at fifteen, when he read Cushing's biography of Osler.)
They related to Brockman as to a guru, and their relationship was marked by all the ambivalence—the reverence,
love, jealousy, and rage—of most such relationships.
("He's a great surgeon, a great neurologist, a great radiologist, a great clinician," said Ken, "but I'd never admit a
bit of it to him.") They knew he'd shaped and inspired their
careers, but they were anxious to see him gone. They felt
he was spending too much time at administration and not
enough in the lab, holding them back by taking too many
interesting cases for himself. But all these offenses, it
seemed to me, were sublimations for a deeper complaint,
the rivalry between them, the fear they felt in his presence. Though they'd worked with him for twelve years,
neither could call him by his first name. His wife was
"Barbara" but he was "Dr. Brockman" or at best "J.B."

Not so long ago, Brockman had phoned Ken and in an unconscious (hard to imagine it conscious with him) attempt to break the ice, announced himself as "Jim." Ken had no idea who he was.

These days much was made about a "generation gap" among neurosurgeons, and surgeons in general, and while a great deal of it was simplistic—or psychological, rather than generational—there were certain differences between generations that spoke of large historical forces. Today's neurosurgery was much more than forty years ahead of the field Brockman had entered in 1940. Technology had shaped it, extended it, and in many ways demystified it. In the early days brain herniation, as Brockman always pointed out, was a constant fear. There was no CAT-scan or angiogram to help plot one's course (though angiography had been invented some time before, it was not yet used routinely), no sophisticated anesthesia, no surgical microscope, no machines for tracking EKG and pulse. A surgeon got in and out as fast as possible, waited for results without technological cover. How could such conditions fail to attract and then reinforce a certain kind of personality? What was demanded was egoism, maximum self-confidence, decisiveness, endless tolerance for failure and risk and anxiety. What was ruled out, absolutely, were minds concerned with ambiguity and abstraction, timidity, fear of the future, and attachment to the past. It was a field that attracted loners and eccentrics and repelled the unadventurous.

Harvey and Ken were far from timid, but they had never known their field without technology. To take a specific but very important example, both were at home with the microscope, at ease with higher magnifications than Brockman liked to use, and this gave them more control in certain procedures. While Brockman was known for his speed, they liked to move slowly, fastidiously. In fact, they prided themselves on patience (hardly a quality one would expect to find—as a source of pride—in an interventionist). Harvey dissected aneurysms after he had clipped them, teased them off the vessels, and tested them for hemorrhage. Not so long ago, that was out of the question; once the clip was installed you withdrew as quickly as possible and hoped your seal was tight.

There were those who thought that the younger people were too cautious (Brockman, by the way, was not one of them; he had nothing but admiration for the new breed of surgeons). Some said they exposed patients to unnecessary strain with long operations and often backed out on tumors when they ought to have gone for more. Certainly there were justifications, these days, for timidity. The consumer movement, unknown in Brockman's day, had taken its toll on medicine (some would say its toll was far too small), and together with inflated medical costs had led to self-criticism and defensiveness among doctors that was unheard of in the forties. Everywhere one looked, there were watchdog groups, controls on expenditures (no equipment was purchased at Osler until approved by four different committees), efficiency studies, and, worst of all, malpractice lawyers. These days nothing inhibited doctors —the younger ones anyhow—like malpractice anxiety. There were said to be case finders circulating in the hospital, spies who sought out patients for lawyers, then took percentage cuts. Recently, a former patient had asked Brockman to justify a new operation on a disk, assure his insurance company that the pain he suffered was not caused by the same disk that had been operated on before (insurance policies did not cover two operations for the same illness). Brockman wrote the company, "It's either a new disk or my mistake that I didn't fix up the other one." He operated again and repaired the disk (a new one, entirely unrelated to the previous operation). The patient walked out of the hospital cured, then sued him for $100,-000.

Though Brockman paid $30,000 a year for malpractice insurance and had five cases (none justified, according to Ken) pending against him, he wasn't really disturbed about the situation. Caution wasn't in his nature, for one thing, and for another, he knew his reputation would carry him a long way in court. For younger people it was another story. A serious case could destroy a doctor's reputation, and the more difficult the surgery attempted, the more likely it was that one would make mistakes or, in their absence, be accused of them. How could a surgeon ignore this pressure or resist the tendency it generated to be overcautious?

Although Harvey and Ken enjoyed the authority and status and the macho image of neurosurgeons, although they worked as hard as the Boss and were equally addicted to the operating room, they weren't the solitary eccentrics of Brockman's generation but rather respectable, hard-working professionals, members of a collective. During college and medical school, Brockman had been an organizer of the Abraham Lincoln Brigade. In fact, he was on the verge of going to Spain to fight against Franco when a superior discouraged him ("You can do more for society as a living physician than as a dead communist"). One could not imagine that sort of radicalism in either Harvey or Ken.

There was glamour too in those days which, though still present, was diminishing all the time. It used to be that if you were good at an operation, you were known for it throughout the world. Harvey and Ken, both equal to anyone at certain difficult procedures, would admit that twenty-five or thirty others could do what they did as well. As Ken explained it, "Neurosurgery used to be like flying single-engine planes into uncharted territory. Nowadays we've got maps, radar, twice as much fuel as we need, all sorts of backup protection. We're flying Seven-forty-sevens." And Harvey put it like this: "They were cowboys in the old days. They rode their horses into the sunset, shot from the hip. We've got much too much to do with our time to spend it on a horse."

After lunch, I walked Harvey and Ken down the hall to the operating rooms, then headed for the ward. As I waited for the elevator, Marvin Welsh—his head bandaged now—was wheeled through the swinging doors toward the recovery room, passing the patient Harvey had scheduled for this afternoon. He was a twenty-five-year-old man with an AVM, a street-wise tough guy, furious because they'd kept him waiting in the hall.

"Listen, man," he said to Harvey, "how much longer you gonna keep me lying here?"

"Not too long, I hope," Harvey said. "We'll be ready for you soon."

"Soon? What does that mean, soon?"

"It means, well, not too long."

"That ain't good enough. I want to know exactly."

"I can't tell you exactly. They've got to get the room ready."

"Tell me exactly, motherfucker, or I'm gettin' the fuck outa here."

Harvey glared at him and began an answer but thought better of it. The last I saw of them, as I stepped on the elevator, Harvey was staring at the wall in disbelief. Thinking, I guess, that today would be like yesterday. Myself, I was thinking that it took no small amount of courage to insult a man who was about to open up your head.

The neurosurgical ward was sixteen rooms on the ninth floor: two singles, ten doubles, four quadruples. Rates at this time ranged from $140 per day for singles to $90 for quads, but according to administration the cost of keeping patients exceeded that by at least 25 percent. Most rooms —and treatment—were covered by insurance, and this had

created an inflationary spiral that many had observed and
none had solved. Since insurance programs seldom covered outpatient therapy, doctors were often forced to
admit patients who might have remained at home. This
created a room shortage, increased expenses, and inevita-
bly increased insurance premiums. The contradiction was
typical of modern medicine, one of many reasons why its
costs have increased much more rapidly than those in
other sectors of the economy.

Measured by its function, the ward was so lacking in
melancholy that it often struck me as surreal. Floors were
ivory-colored linoleum squares, walls were orange and yellow, lights hidden and benevolent. Along each wall were
aluminum rails for patients who required them, and at the
end of the hall was the cheerful Visitors' Lounge where
Bryan and David held their weekly meetings. Windows
were huge, sunlight plentiful, sound muted. There were
many days when I was glad to return here, more than one
when I was shocked to remember why people checked into
these rooms.

Rooms with northern exposure had a view of the river
and the highway and the footpath—used mostly these
days by runners—that ran beside it. George Tinker, a former runner who would never run again, would often stand
there watching the runners below, dealing, as he put it,
with the movies in his mind. "Jealousy, anger, memories,
dreams, I might as well get used to them." The week
before, during evening rounds, while Brockman was examining a patient whose tumor he'd removed, President
Carter drove up the highway in a motorcade and everyone
rushed to the window. "He's okay," said Brockman, returning to his patient. "He's done a good job." And the
patient: "If you ask me, he's nothing compared to you."

The nurses' station was in the middle of the floor, halfway between the two banks of elevators, and behind it was
the meeting room where the Boss met with his staff and

held meetings such as the one he'd had with Charlie White and his family. Hanging on a hook next to the bulletin board was the plastic card the nurses used with patients who could not speak. It had silhouettes for messages, needs the patients could not express: a knife and fork, a toilet, a glass of water, a radio, a television. Patients who could understand this chart were more or less in business. If not, a larger sensitivity was required of the staff, but that was less of a problem than one would think. Good nurses often know what patients need before they know it themselves.

There were several plaques on the wall, brass plates on mahogany frames, the sort of testimonials that corporations give longtime employees when they retire. THANK YOU, said one, FOR MAKING A DIFFICULT TIME LESS DIFFICULT. And another: FROM THE CONLINS, OF TULSA, OKLAHOMA, TO THE NURSES AND DOCTORS ON THE NINTH FLOOR AT OSLER MEMORIAL: THANK YOU FOR YOUR KINDNESS DURING OUR DAYS OF GRIEF. There was a postcard from Florida—*To let you know that Viola Croft is still alive!*—and a notice from the operating floor—PLEASE MAKE SURE THAT NAIL POLISH IS REMOVED BEFORE PATIENTS ARE SENT DOWN FOR SURGERY—and finally a bizarre bulletin from the rehabilitation department concerning (I think) a recent advance in mobility research:

> Myoelectric and biomechanical data generated during motion against resistance, recorded simultaneously, constitute a biomechanical profile which permits objective evaluation of changes in functional capacity resulting from therapy and/or modifications of man-equipment interfaces.

Leaving the elevator, I met Sister Callahan, and we walked together down the hall. She was a stout, white-

haired woman with blue eyes and very broad shoulders, a
sixty-two-year-old nun who was born two blocks from the
hospital and educated at the same Catholic school in the
neighborhood where, after she'd become a nun, she had
taught English and eventually became principal. For the
last twenty-five years, she had lived at a convent next door
to the school. Two years ago, Brockman had removed part
(subtotal excision, they called it) of a large malignant
tumor which had compromised her language and memory
and finished her as a teacher. Since he liked her a great
deal and hated to see her vegetate in the convent while
waiting for her tumor to return, he had invited her to work
here as a volunteer, hang around the ward, and share with
other patients the miraculous equanimity she seemed to
feel about her condition. It was a measure of his creativity
as a physician that he had chosen what was, for her, an
ideal form of therapy. I met no other doctor at the hospital
who would have thought of such a thing, or done it if he
had.

She arrived mornings at seven thirty and hung around
until six or seven at night, or until her strength gave out,
doing favors for the patients and nurses (joyous to go for
a magazine or a candy bar), talking with anyone who
sought her out—nothing essential, but people missed her
when she didn't show up and felt better when she did. She
had a lot of trouble with words, calling the Catholic church,
for instance, "that place uptown," and the hospital, "that
little blue thing," but she laughed at herself, and that
quality—in combination with her deficit—made her a sort
of hero with the patients. When she said, "Take it easy,
you can do it," it wasn't because she'd learned to say it in
school. There were certain patients who terrified everyone
on the staff, but Sister Callahan could sit with them for
hours at a time. Lately, she'd begun to regress, stammer-
ing more and dragging her right foot. It was clear even
without a scan that the tumor had resumed its growth, but

she seemed indifferent to her prospects. If anything, her calm increased. "It will come back," she assured me once, apropos of nothing. (Needless to say, a lot was said around this ward apropos of nothing.) "What will come back?" I said. And she: "Everything. And if it doesn't, it's just a matter of pride."

As usual, the nurses had rolled Tony Kirtz to the station, where they could keep an eye on him. Like Sister Callahan, he had a glioma, but his was in the hypothalamic region and it had affected him as it does a lot of patients, making him belligerent and unpredictable and frequently obscene. The Boss had taken a shot at his tumor two weeks ago, getting maybe 75 percent, and now, with radiation, his prospects weren't so bad. He was sixty-eight, a watchmaker before his illness. His tumor had announced itself in a Chinese restaurant when, according to his daughter, he fell into his chop suey. Before surgery, he'd spoken English, French, and his native Polish, but now he'd lost French altogether, and most of his English. He had spent most of last week screaming in Polish, which no one on the ward could understand, but this week, as the swelling in his brain diminished, his English had improved. The nurses kept him at the station, tied with a strap to his wheelchair, because three times he'd gotten out of bed and tried to run away and because he had been grabbing their breasts and exposing himself to the wife of his roommate, who happened to be Andy March. "My husband in a coma," she said, "and I've got to deal with that?"

Tony liked to talk, and he kept a wry grin all the time. He'd point his finger at you when you came down the hall, demanding, "Where are you, young fella?" and if you answered, he'd rail at you in Polish. This morning, as Sister Callahan and I approached, he varied it just a little. "And you? And you? Where are you?"

"I'm in the hospital," I said. "Same as you, Tony."

"No, you're not. I want to know where you really are."

Sister Callahan put her arm on his shoulder. "Listen, Tony, you be a good boy," she began, but he reached for her skirt and pulled on it as if he meant to tear it off.

She was so little bothered that I thought he must have done it before. Stepping back calmly, she eased herself beyond his reach. "Oh, boy!" she cried. "What in the world do you think you're doing?"

"That's my business," Tony said.

"Your business nothing. You're a bad boy. Why don't you behave yourself?"

"Why should I?" Tony said. And waving his hand as if to dismiss us, he gave the same excuse he offered Mrs. March when she berated him for exposing himself: "I'm a paying tenant."

Unlike the neurology ward on the eighth floor, there was rapid turnover here. George Tinker was gone already, Rosie was gone, Peter Fleischman was gone. Mostly, patients were treated and dismissed. Long-term cases for the most part were those like Raymond Dreyer, who required radiation and could not manage on an outpatient basis (he was from the Midwest and had no relatives here), or patients with back or pain problems—operable or inoperable—that required bed rest and rehabilitation. Many of these should not have been here at all. They came on the possibility that they were surgical, then often grew dependent on the hospital and stayed until the Boss had to force them out. "She's leaving Friday," he said once. "I don't care if we have to get a moving van and roll her bed into it."

The transience and discontinuity were sometimes disconcerting. You would get very close to certain patients and feel bereft when they were gone, develop a sense of community during the week and discover on Monday that you knew no one on the floor. Nor did it help that you were happy for patients that they were going home. Everyone got attached to people who stayed around awhile, and a room where everything gelled like that became a sanctuary, like a bar where you knew your friends were drinking.

At that time Room 934 was my retreat. Raymond Dreyer lived there, and a gentleman named Dr. Chardan, a sixty-five-year-old physician who gave platitudinous, inspirational sermons to his roommates and anyone else who would listen, and Mr. Sedgwick, a professional fisherman who had had a heart attack on the table while Harvey was clipping his aneurysm, and Arthur Rodgers, a former accountant ("I used to be what you might call an accountant") who had a problem similar to Mr. Dreyer's. Since all but Sedgwick suffered urinary incontinence, I had been invited there—"Any day at noon"—for bedwetting competition. What they meant was that at noon the nurse would total up the number of pajamas each had used during the previous twenty-four hours. I never found out whether the winner was the one who'd used the most or least, and I'm not sure they found out either.

Arthur and Raymond were watching television (soaps) when I arrived, and Sedgwick and Chardan were sitting by the window in their wheelchairs, watching traffic below and continuing an argument they'd been having since they met. I asked Arthur if he wanted to talk, but there was no competing with the television. From Raymond I got the same response. TVs in general were rarely turned off up here, even when the doctors came for rounds. Each bed had a set of its own, attached to the wall with a telescoping arm that allowed you to swing it around until it was right against your face. There were earphones, but they were seldom used. You could hear four different channels at times in a quadruple room like this. At night, when rounds were finished and visiting hours done, lights turned down, and meal trays stacked outside the door, television was often the only sound you heard. Imagine gunshots here, commercials. Imagine canned laughter. An aphasic patient like Raymond Dreyer watching "As the World Turns."

I was disappointed that Arthur wouldn't talk to me. I

had followed him closely since his operation, from the terrible aphasia which he'd endured in the first few days, to his present status, which permitted clarity as well as malapropism of the sort that made one think aphasia might not be a disintegration of language but a reinvention. "I've a bounty of mementos," he said, when he showed me photos of his children, and—about a nurse he didn't like—"She is not full of wonder." When he wanted quiet, he asked for "queer," and, speaking of his postoperative problems, "I walked a lot of clods."

I waited a bit to see if he would talk, but he continued to ignore me until I walked away. Then, "Wait," he cried. "My hand!" He was holding up his weak hand and wanted me to test it. The right hand was often plegic after surgery (or stroke) on the left side of the brain, and it was often the most dramatic measure of improvement to feel it getting better. Many patients asked you, as Arthur did now, to let them squeeze your thumb so you could evaluate their grip.

"It's stronger," I said. "No doubt about it."

Arthur beamed with pleasure, and then he began to weep. Brain damage, of almost any sort, can often make one labile; patients can sob one minute and laugh the next, changing so quickly that sometimes they seem to be doing both at the same time. Still squeezing my hand, tears streaming down his cheeks, Arthur had nevertheless returned to his television. I stroked his hand for a moment, then disengaged. "Thanks, pal!" he cried, as I walked away. "Try me tomorrow!"

Chardan and Sedgwick were anxious for me to join them, each looking to get me on his side against the other. Chardan leaned toward inspiration, believed in the power of positive thinking, too much of which—unless you met someone as intransigent as Sedgwick—could not be mustered in this ward. He had been a practicing physician (an internist) until a tumor had appeared on his spinal cord, paralyzing him from the neck down, restricting his breathing, and—by his own estimate—traumatizing him with fear. He wore a collar on his neck now ("What happens," he asked Harvey, "when it's removed?" "Your head falls off"), but the operation had been a complete success, and having come through his fear, he felt cleansed, reborn, hungry to share his joy in life with others.

Sedgwick thought him completely out of his mind. He considered his own operation a foolish mistake, an act of weakness, and though he enjoyed Chardan, he resented his efforts to convince him otherwise. An aneurysm had brought Sedgwick here, but he had a history of vascular problems and arteriosclerosis which had made him nearly blind and given him headaches and seizures for years. Though aware of the aneurysm, he had resisted surgery because his condition was hereditary, and he thought it wiser and more practical to accept his destiny than seek to circumvent it. His mother, who had suffered from similar problems, had spent the last eleven years of her life in a coma, vegetating, with her arms crossed on her chest (Sedgwick swore that when she died and her arms were lifted, there were holes in her chest where her fists had been), in the back bedroom of the family house. Far greater than his fear of death was his fear of ending up like her. He had finally allowed his wife and children to sell him on surgery, but then he'd had a heart attack on the table, and now, after his surgery, none of his symptoms had improved. The way he saw it, he'd not only suffered for nothing but increased the likelihood that he would suffer more. "Positive thinking" struck him as another con to add to the many he'd endured.

"Please sit down," Chardan said to me. "This man needs some encouragement, and maybe you're the one to give it to him."

"Why do I need encouragement?" Sedgwick said. "What good's that gonna do me?"

"Don't pay any attention to him. He's feeling sorry for himself today."

"Sorry? Maybe I am, maybe I am. And maybe you can tell me why I shouldn't. Can you give me one good reason why a man in my condition shouldn't feel sorry for himself?"

"Why should you not?"

Chardan had the voice of an evangelist. I never figured out whether he had always spoken like this—a country preacher with a tremolo in the lower register—or whether his illness had induced it. His tumor had caused him to lose his voice for several weeks before surgery, so it was not impossible that these electronic sounds (it was easy to mistake him for the television) were pathological. Whatever their cause, their effect was melodramatic and irresistible. Since he was a doctor and thus could back up what he said with some experience, he carried more weight on the ward than anyone else except the surgeons themselves.

"Why should you not?" repeated Chardan. "Because you have life, sir. Life! You have recovered from one of the most serious diseases in our lexicon. With luck you'll be able to ponder your experience for a long time. Though, of course, you'd be well advised not to ponder it. Look at you, sir! Your senses are not one bit impaired! You are aware of everything! Your only problem is that you're doing what we all do, wallowing in your fear. Take yourself in hand, Mr. Sedgwick! Look at what you have instead of what you haven't."

Sometimes this sermon worked (Arthur, for one, adored it), but Sedgwick was unmoved. He shook his head while Chardan spoke, then leaned close to him and whispered, "Others up here may buy that shit, Chardan, but not me, no sir, not me. Surgery was the biggest mistake I ever made. I had to grab onto a couple more years of a perfectly good life! What did I care if my brain fell apart? I live on the waterfront! I coulda jumped and ended it clean!"

"Ah, Mr. Sedgwick, wake up to yourself. You're afraid of falling into your mother's basket."

"You're damned right I am! Who wants to end up a vegetable? Take every bit of your family's money, drain 'em dry, make the doctors rich, for what? For what? Why should we grab onto every last little bit of life? I say, take what you have and be happy with it. Don't listen to these assholes who say you should live forever."

I listened to them long enough to know that neither would move the other, then went off down the hall. Dr. Chardan had conveyed a message that another long-term patient, Allan Benjamin, had urgent business to discuss with me, so I went to look for him.

In the hall I came upon Sister Callahan, walking arm-in-arm with Clemencia Lopez on their daily stroll around the ward. It was one of the sister's chores to encourage Clemencia in her exercise. A stroke patient in her early sixties, admitted to the hospital because they were considering an anastomosis as a means of bringing blood to the deficient regions of her brain, Clemencia was stubborn and recalcitrant, hated anything that got her out of bed, and only Sister Callahan could make her move. She was a Cuban woman with keen, intimidating eyes and—if I read her correctly—a private sense of humor. Almost everything she said was related to the Cuban political situation. What she insinuated mostly was that she was a member of the secret police—of which country she wouldn't say—and that her visit to the hospital was related to her work.

Since her right hand, as a result of her stroke, was still in a sling, she took my hand in her left.

"Clemencia has been asking about you," Sister Callahan said.

"Asking what? What was it you wanted to know, Clemencia?"

She looked over her shoulder, shutting one eye suspiciously. "I'm not at liberty to say."

"Why not?"

"I told you, I can't say. I am in a delicate position. I am for Fidel and against him, you understand?"

"Of course I understand. I won't say another word."

She studied me fiercely, shutting one eye again. "Do you know anything?"

"No, nothing. Do you?"

"I do and I don't. About the leaders, I'm not talking. There's good and there's bad, but I won't say which is which."

I took her hand again. "Okay, Clemencia. Take it easy!"

"Yeah!" she said, smiling. "You take it easy too!"

I found Allan Benjamin in the Visitors' Lounge, sitting opposite Marvin Welsh's parents, who were waiting for him to come upstairs from the recovery room. Benjamin, at the time, was the ward's principal guardian of the conviction that Brockman was God, although there were others who, as one might imagine, were anxious to contest him. Ten days before, the Boss had removed the second acoustic tumor which Allan's brain had produced in the last eight years. Since Brockman had done the operation in five hours and the first surgeon (as prominent as Brockman) had required sixteen, Allan was a concrete advertisement of Brockman's speed and dexterity, and he never tired of propagandizing for him.

Acoustic tumors are tedious affairs, and their surgical treatment sometimes involves complex psychological issues. The seventh cranial (or facial) nerve is often affected, and surgeons have to weigh the dangers of the tumor against the cosmetic ramifications of its removal. As Brockman explained it, "You have to get enough tumor to relieve pressure on the brain stem and the cerebellum, as well as any hydrocephalus it may cause. Then you have to ask yourself, If I take the whole tumor, will I damage the facial nerve? And then: Is it worth that, or better to leave some inside? You know you've helped the patient, but sometimes you also know you have to get more to keep him alive. The best thing is to talk it over with patients beforehand and let them decide for themselves . . . that is, if you know the story yourself before you go in."

Needless to say, such decisions, involving as they do a choice between life and vanity, often call forth ambivalent response.

"I did a forty-year-old woman last year who was married to a thirty-five-year-old airline pilot. Sat down with her and explained the whole thing, all the dangers, all the possible side effects, and so forth. She thought about it maybe ten seconds, then she said, 'Leave some if you have to. No way I'm gonna hold onto my husband with a paralyzed face.' "

Since Benjamin had made the other choice, he had lost a good deal of his facial control. The right side of his mouth sagged and he spoke with great difficulty, drooling heavily. Once, perhaps, his face had been handsome, but it was flaccid now, devoid of energy. Since he did not like to wear his postsurgical watch cap, his scar was visible and grotesque, the black sutures curling off his scalp like insects. He was a football coach by profession, married, living in the suburbs. His teenage son, like George Tinker's, had underlined his illness by beating him at tennis.

What Allan wanted was to tap my secret line to Brockman. Like a lot of patients, he had endless imaginary conversations with him, considered him indeed an intimate friend, but—also like a lot of patients—he was too much in awe to address him about anything not absolutely essential. The first "urgency" on his mind today was Brockman's smoking habits. Being obsessed himself with physical health, a fanatic especially about cigarettes, Allan thought it an outrage that a man of Brockman's stature should set such a bad example.

"Tell me, how can a man of such genius, such knowledge

of the human body, subject himself to the insult of to-
bacco?"

"Why don't you ask him yourself?"

"He's too busy. I am after all just a patient, but he's
. . . well, he's too busy for people like me."

I had spoken with Benjamin before and I was beginning
to realize that this conversation, like our others, was
mostly a subterfuge to provide him with a listener. Certain
patients who had no mental deficits could become obsessive and clinging and not a little domineering. The trauma
of surgery combined with all this empty time: what could
make a man more infantile more quickly, or bring out more
insecurity?

The second "urgency" was a painkilling machine, invented by a friend of his, which he felt the Boss should
know about. It was an electrical device which attached to
the muscle and worked, he assured me, as well as Novo-
caine. Who could say what miracles a machine like that
might work if brought to neurosurgery?

Next he had a complaint, a certain physical therapist
down in Rehab who enraged him every morning by re-
questing that, while walking, he "swish his hips" a little.
Though the purpose of this (which Benjamin should have
been able to deduce) was to increase the mobility in his
pelvic region, he considered it an insult to his masculinity,
and he wanted the Boss to reprimand her. "I don't know
how you feel about such things, but . . . all my life I've been
an athlete. Swishing is not my style." There followed an
account of his athletic history, a description of his tennis
game, his handball, his high-school basketball and football.
"Only one hundred and forty pounds, but do you know
where I played? Right guard! I moved men that out-
weighed me by fifty pounds. I was a hitter, that's what
everyone said. Afraid of nothing."

It wasn't comfortable, feeling bored and sympathetic at
the same time, but the contradiction was one to which you

grew accustomed on the ward. I knew what he needed now, what it meant for him to speak with me, who was part of the Boss's entourage, and God knows, nostalgia for youth and athletics was hardly uncommon up here. But sympathy wasn't always enough to make one compassionate. On long days like this one, there would often come a time when tolerance deserted me and patients, no matter how much I sought to be sympathetic, became obnoxious. Some, if you let them, would consume you. See them in context, and you could forgive them anything, but when you were tired, and sated on the pain, the context could disappear and all you'd see was their self-absorption. Many felt guilty when they got to this anger, but guilt was a cul-de-sac. The best it could do was make you patronize the patient with false compassion, and the worst—well, it could make you hollow and supercilious, make you treat them as objects. The anger was nothing less than your instinct to survive. What can you give to anyone if you can't give in to that?

The sun was level with the windows, dropping toward the river. Outside, where I had not been since six thirty that morning, one of the first days of spring was bathing the city with visions of health and good fortune. It struck me that I had rarely looked out these windows, that these halls and the world outside were separated by an absolute demarcation. Even if one looked, one did not actually see. From here the "real" world was flat and two-dimensional, as if the windows were a television screen.

I felt an overwhelming urge to leave the hospital, take a walk in the park, circulate among people who had other things besides their bodies on their mind—people who, like all except the brain-damaged, can forget sometimes that they have brains. I said good-bye to Allan, took the elevator down to the lobby, and headed for the revolving door that connected the hospital to reality. There was an ambulance outside, a patient parked beside it on a stretcher.

There were also signs of health. A nurse sat on the steps with an ice-cream cone, and a young couple sprawled on the grass, laughing as though life had nothing but joy in store for them. Already beginning the curious transformation that occurred every day when I left the hospital, the radical mind-shift that made the place almost impossible to remember as soon as it was left behind, I pushed through the door and came face to face with Brockman, who had just stepped out of a cab.

"Where are you going?" he said.

"I don't know," I said. "I thought maybe for a walk."

"A walk? It's only four fifteen!"

"I know, but I'm a little tired."

"Come on," he said, taking my arm and turning me around. "I'll buy you a cup of coffee. Lots of interesting stuff to see this afternoon."

8

Inappropriate Smiles

And so it resumed, the power and its management, the intervention, the perpetual motion, and, most of all, the energy that could be generated by Brockman and the hospital in combination, the sense that the pain was under control, reality subservient to skill. Within five minutes of joining him, I'd forgotten my fatigue.

We went first to check out Marvin Welsh in the recovery room (no problems so far), then to radiology to read the new angiograms, then to the cafeteria for the coffee he'd promised and a couple of candy bars, and finally back to the eighth floor, neurology, for the weekly conference where neurologists and neurosurgeons reviewed the problem cases on their wards.

As we left radiology, we passed the CAT-scan room and, finding one of his patients on the table, Brockman gave me yet another glimpse of the magical technology he had at his disposal. Since the machine provided, in addition to Polaroid prints, a videoscan which could be read directly on a television set, he turned some switches on a monitor and searched out the pictures he required: "slices" of the patient's brain which the computer had assembled from the

28,000 readings the camera collected. The patient was a middle-aged man who'd had a tumor removed three months before, and the purpose of the scan was to determine if it was coming back. We could see him on the table through a window in this, the control room, his head in a rubber collar, the scanner moving slowly around him. On the TV screen "slices" appeared until one displayed, like a puff of black smoke, the tumor. "Shit," said the Boss. "He's not doing well at all."

Neurology Conference was just beginning when we arrived, the room already packed with attendants, residents, interns, and medical students from both the neurology and neurosurgery departments. The first patient had just been introduced. Brockman took the seat reserved for him beside Reynolds Clarke, the chief of neurology, lit up a cigarette, and studied the patient, who was sitting at the front of the room while a resident stood behind her, reciting the sort of litany which by now was so familiar: "This is a sixty-two-year-old right-handed woman who presented last week with episodes of intermittent confusion, pus in her left ear, and—one day prior to admission—severe aphasia."

Conference was obviously critical to the work, a chance to review mistakes and share new information, educate the younger people, and—most important, perhaps—define the community that existed here among staff members. In addition to this meeting, there were three others held on a weekly basis: one for neurosurgeons and neuroradiologists; one conducted by the neurologists, which neurosurgeons were expected to attend; and one called Brain Cutting, or Pathology Conference, where pathologists presented the brains of patients who'd died during the week or microscopic slides of tissue that surgeons had removed from patients who were still alive. Another meeting, a monthly affair, was a sort of moment of truth for the surgeons alone. It was called Death Conference or—if outsiders were present—Mortality Conference, and it consisted of a review of all the patients who'd died during the previous month.

Conferences differed in atmosphere as well as content, and taken together, they offered a multimedia spectacle which, on subjects one had thought to be consistent, rivaled Proust in shifting points of view. At Neurosurgery Conference on Friday afternoon, videotapes of difficult operations (such as the one Brockman expected would soothe Ken Beck's ego by being this week's star) were presented, mistakes and solutions discussed, surprises shared. "We got behind the optic nerve and found the cyst, but just when we thought we were done, we saw this mass of tumor—see it there?—behind the cyst and had to go after it." "I was moving the tumor back and forth with my bayonet and suddenly—watch this!—it popped out in one piece, purple as a plum." The mood here was what I'd come to expect from neurosurgeons, much joking and laughter, very little boredom or restlessness or fatigue. Descriptions were economical and unambiguous, concrete and merciless in their exactitude. "We approached the lesion through a Faulkner flap. In between the two branches of the vein of Labbé we made our incision, as you see. Then we bluntly dissected the white matter." "She was taken to the O.R., where we simply reelevated the previous bone flap, opened the dura inferiorly, did a partial right frontal lobectomy, as had been done on the previous occasion, then retracted the brain and readily exposed the optic nerve." "After his lumbar puncture he complained of headaches and was told to lie down. Five minutes later there was a commotion in the room, and he was noted to be banging his arm on the side rail, pointing to his plegic right side, which had been fine before. In front of our eyes he became decerebrate on the right side."

The procession was endless and never undramatic, but, as always with surgery, the problems, however vast, were finite, convergent, pointing toward, if not arriving at, clear-cut solution or failure, like a game in which the bottom line will always be clear on the scoreboard. Neurology Conference was less like a game than a seminar. In fact, the two conferences differed almost exactly as their constituents did. The neurological material was interesting enough, but the diseases were intransigent, diffuse, and usually incurable. Instead of videotapes, there were figures on the blackboard, statistics, test results. Sometimes the entire meeting was given over to a lecture on new research in one particular area, like stroke or parkinsonism. I never saw anyone sleeping at a neurosurgery conference, but it wasn't rare here to find half a dozen nodding off. Excitement was available, of course, but you had to work for it. If you didn't, the boredom was oppressive.

It was possible to hear the same patient discussed at both the neurology and the neurosurgery conferences, then later at Brain Cutting and, if he didn't make it, at Death Conference too. Patients were usually admitted and worked up by the neurologists, who'd present their cases at Neurology Conference to determine, among other things, whether they were surgical. If they were, tapes of their operations might be shown a couple of weeks later at Neurosurgery Conference. And then, if a tumor was removed successfully, you might see slides of it the following week at Brain Cutting; or, if the patient died, a slice of his brain, bathed in formalin and tagged with a red identity card: BRAIN 2339.

Brain Cutting was a trip in the direction of the Grand Guignol, a reduction to the other side of zero. Tumor slides were beautiful, lyrical, hallucinatory birds or insects, aerial photographs of deserts or mountain ranges, visions of the microcosm or the macrocosm, images to feed your dreams. While they were displayed, pathologists and surgeons took turns describing them, surgeons summarizing

the patients, pathologists the tumors. Steeped in detachment and glib as newscasters, their voices accompanied
the light show like the sound track of a surrealist film.
"Usually with grade-five astrocytomas you don't see this
sort of configuration, but the cell density is consistent with
that diagnosis." If patients were dead and their brains or
spinal cords presented, they were passed around the room
on yellow plastic lunch trays. Dreadful as it sounds, there
was something benign and anticlimactic about this procedure, as if—now that the mind-matter paradox was finally
resolved and the brain merely a piece of meat on a yellow
tray—it lacked all power and resonance. Devoid of its ambiguity, it was also devoid of mystery. You'd touch it and
smell it, waiting for cracks in your perception, some seizure of fear or flash of intuition, but nothing came. It was
just a smelly piece of brown and white meat, a bit like a
veal cutlet, with a texture like foam rubber and the shape
(really beautiful) of a butterfly. It made a lot more sense
to speak of it aesthetically than to consider it as the organ
that might once have made aesthetics possible.

Death Conference, of course, offered another kind of
reduction, another shift in the kaleidoscope, this one retro-
spective like Brain Cutting but denied the luxury of its
fragmentation. It was the long shot you got here, a quick
summary of the denouement, a peek over the shoulder at
the last dark corridor, but unlike Brain Cutting, the brain
under consideration was yet haunted by the being it had
once inhabited. Exclusively for neurosurgeons, Death
Conference was held on the first Monday of every month,
and its mood, perhaps because it was held in the evening,
was relaxed and informal, more at odds with the material
discussed than any other meeting. Sandwiches and soft
drinks and beer were laid out in a lovely spread next to the
slide projector, and while everyone ate, catastrophes were
reconsidered and debated so that their causes could be
ascertained and the principal question—avoidable or not?

—be laid to rest. In addition to the sandwiches, everyone was provided with a sheet that summarized the cases in medicalese, the amazing language of all the conferences which seemed here to emerge in its ultimate flower.

> Forty-seven-year-old Caucasian male
> readmitted for recurrent acoustic neuroma
> initially operated a year prior to admission.
> Did well postoperatively for one year but
> began to have gait difficulty, lethargy,
> anisocoria, nystagmus in all directions.
> Left-central facial weakness, dysmetria,
> bilateral spasticity with hyperreflexia
> bilaterally, bilateral papilledema and
> confusion.

One could actually put the case together from the sheet, but it was a bit more palatable to listen to the resident in charge of the presentation, who read from the sheet and interjected salient material: "On the fourth day subsequent to admission, he was taken to the O.R. for total removal of a right-cerebello-pontine angle recurrent neuroma with profuse bleeding at the final stage of tumor removal." (Translation: he hemorrhaged on the table.)

Occasionally, when death was unexpected, as with this patient, questions came from the floor. And since the surgeon, in this case, was the Boss, a certain euphemistic strategy was required.

"Unusual, isn't it, Boss, to get the artery at this point?"

"Ah, shit, it was just a technical error. We were pulling with a pituitary forceps, thinking we had it clear, but there must've been a loop of tumor hooked around the artery. No way to see the sonofabitch at all."

Usually the resident read no more, and they proceeded at once to the next case. They had an average of ten to twenty deaths a month to process (nearly all of them re-

sulting from acute illness that surgery had not reversed),
and there was seldom time for all the information on the
sheet. I offer it here because, like the surgeons' dictations
in the locker room, these summaries were unique in their
capacity to reduce illness to its most banal (and "manageable") components and so to reveal the particular mechanics of the surgeon's mind, the psychology that made it
possible to deal with this sort of horror day after day.

> Day five. Vital signs stable. Patient
> unconscious. Pupils bilaterally fixed and
> dilated. Minimal response to pain. On
> respirator. Remained in this state and expired
> on May 22 (day eight).
>
> Clinical diagnosis: Right recurrent
> cerebello-pontine angle tumor. s/p resection.
> s/p respirator therapy.
>
> Pathology diagnosis: nerve sheath tumor. s/p
> resection VIII sheath tumor, R. Subarachnoid
> hematoma cerebrum and cerebellum, bilateral,
> recent. Infarct, hemorrhagic, extensive, brain
> stem and cerebellar hemisphere, R, recent;
> cerebral edema, diffuse. Arteriosclerosis
> cerebri, moderate. s/p respirator therapy, four
> days.

Neurology Conference, the one we entered now, was of
all the conferences unique for its "humanity," way at the
other end of the spectrum from Brain Cutting or Death
Conference. Living patients were presented here, disease
that might be curable, brains which somehow, on some
level, were interrelated with the mind. The purpose of the
meeting was to work out, step by step, a collective diagnosis and a consensus on the treatment that was required.

The first patient was Mrs. Lyons, a small woman with
curvature of the spine (not related to her illness), her blond

hair so neatly coiffed and dyed that she looked as if she were made up for this occasion. Since she'd caught a bad cold three weeks before her admission, and her symptoms were diffuse, her problem could have been anything from a brain abscess (which can arise from infections in other parts of the body) to a tumor. In the usual manner, the resident in charge, a brooding, distracted fellow named Lamar, began the presentation by summarizing her condition—reflexes, visual fields, hearing, and the results of her spinal tap (the composition of her cerebrospinal fluid). Mrs. Lyons sat with head bowed during this recitation, as if too timid to face the audience, but when Lamar asked her how she felt, she raised her head and smiled happily.

"Thank you, doctor. Very nice to now."

Lamar turned to the audience and repeated her words. " 'Very nice to now.' As you see, she's still aphasic, but we think she's getting better. Yesterday her answers were garbled."

Reynolds Clarke interrupted him. He was a tall, white-haired man with the air of a police interrogator. In contrast to Brockman, who'd recommended him for his job and considered him a close personal friend, Clarke was known as a man who kept a rigid schedule, arriving for work at eight thirty and leaving at five, no matter what situations he encountered. Since he was also, as I've noted, one of those rare neurologists who were sympathetic to the idea of aggressive neurosurgery, he was an ideal complement for the Boss, and their relationship was one of the principal reasons for the department's success.

"All right, Dr. Lamar," Clarke said, "we know she's aphasic. But wouldn't we like to know a little more about her aphasia? What else might you ask her now?"

Lamar was stumped. "I don't know, sir. I wanted merely to demonstrate the speech—"

"Demonstrate?" Clarke was disgusted. "What good is that? There's all different kinds of aphasia! Does she know she's made a mistake? Is she aware of what she said? Mrs. Lyons, tell me please, when you said, 'Very nice to now,' did it sound correct to you?"

"No, sir," said Mrs. Lyons.

"There," Clarke said. "Now we know a bit about her aphasia. Sometimes patients babble without awareness and sometimes they're very concerned with locating the proper words. It's not enough to indicate aphasia. We have to know what kind of aphasia we're dealing with if it's to help us locate the problem in her brain. Go on, Dr. Lamar."

Lamar was tall and thin, a frightened-looking man with thick, connected eyebrows and a habit of standing on one foot while scratching his ankle with the toe of the other. He had an automatic smile which, however much it may have plagued him at other times, was especially unfortunate now, since Mrs. Lyons had one too and it was his job to mark it as a symptom.

"Note, please, her inappropriate smile. According to her husband, this expression was not present until onset of her symptoms last week."

It was difficult to watch him without being embarrassed, almost pained, by his self-consciousness. It was especially disconcerting because of the authority he was expected to wield. He was like a child stretching for a cookie jar just out of reach. I had seen him present patients before and always felt the same embarrassment, mostly, I think, because he demonstrated a particular insecurity about the doctor-patient relationship, the fragility of the line between the examiner and the examined, the luck of the draw that gave some people white jackets and placed others before them as objects. Watching him now, I remembered the first such demonstration I'd had, from an elderly neurologist at a hospital where I worked as a volunteer. He had just given me a wonderful lecture on the difference between short-term and long-term memory and as he stood up to leave, he said, "I won't be in the hospital tomorrow,

but I'll be here Wednesday if you want to talk some more."
I walked him to the elevator, and as he turned away, I said,
"All right, I'll see you Wednesday." "Wednesday?" he
said. "I won't be here Wednesday. I'm on vacation for the
next two weeks."

Lamar tested Mrs. Lyons in the usual way for logic. "Do
helicopters feed their young?"

"Don't be silly."

"How are a banana and an orange alike?"

"They're not alike."

This answer indicated concrete thinking, one of the common characteristics of brain damage, and it elicited much
discussion: was it a sign of transient confusion or a specific
lesion, and, if the latter, what sort of lesion might it be?

Brockman, who'd been silent until now, pointed a finger
at a neurologist in the front row. "Dr. Gross, what do you
think? Has this lady got a neurological problem?"

"Yes, sir," Gross replied. "I think she does."

"Okay, then. We've got memory loss and confusion and
a bit of concrete thinking. Does that localize it?"

"I'd say yes, yes, it does. It indicates a problem in the
posterior temporal lobe."

"Like hell it does. Memory loss and confusion indicate
diffuse neurological dysfunction, but they have no localiz-
ing value whatsoever." He turned to Clarke. "What do you
think, Reynolds? Where do we go from here?"

"What I'm thinking," Clarke said, "is what about her
ear infection? We've got to link that up with confusion!
Hell, we'd all like to think they're not connected, but
they came on at the same time. There's no way we're
going to keep them apart. Isn't anybody curious why
she has no pain? I know I am! With an ear infection
and all these other symptoms, wouldn't you sure as hell
expect she'd have a headache? Does she have one she
hasn't mentioned? Or is she really without pain? I think
she would have mentioned it, don't you? But if that's

the case, what the hell do we do with her infection? No pain! That blows my mind!''

Clarke questioned several interns, forcing them to eliminate certain conditions and to indicate which tests should now be performed on Mrs. Lyons. It was clear that they'd arrive at nothing conclusive about her case this afternoon. In fact, there was nothing to do about her illness but wait it out, "sit on her," as Brockman put it. Someone suggested an angiogram, but the Boss was against it. "Hell," he said, "she's getting better. Why should we bother her with an angiogram? It might have academic interest, but it makes no sense from a clinical standpoint."

Clarke agreed, suggesting they move on to the next patient. "Thank you for your time, Mrs. Lyons."

"Oh, don't mention it!" cried Mrs. Lyons. She stood up to go as if concluding a performance, not a little disappointed, it seemed to me, that it was over. For all the humiliation attendant on these presentations, most patients enjoyed them, considering it some sort of honor that they'd been chosen to appear.

"Interesting," Brockman said, when the door had closed behind her, and then, to my amazement, "I'd bet my life she'll be okay within a week. It's an abscess. And it's resolving itself."

"I think so too," Clarke said. "We'll give her the memory test in a couple of days, and if she's continued improving we'll send her home. Who's got the next patient?"

There was some rustling of paper and shifting of chairs, a bit of small talk and socializing (Brockman lighting still another cigarette), but the time between patients was so brief that one had little time to process Mrs. Lyons. It was necessary, after all, to learn to relinquish patients as well as attend to them, so her quick replacement by the next patient, a forty-five-year-old man named Philip Beale, was itself a part of the education here. Another resident rose and erased the blackboard, chalked in Beale's essentials

where Mrs. Lyons's had been before, posted new angiograms and CAT-scans, and then, taking from his pocket
one of those packages of index cards they used to keep
notes on patients, read to us of Mr. Beale. Did anyone in
the room remember Mrs. Lyons? Not Brockman, for sure.
He could forget patients the instant he left their rooms.
His attention span was completely pragmatic, no longer or
shorter than it had to be, as much a function of what he
could forget as what he could remember.

Philip Beale was a lot more complicated and a lot less
pleasant to face than Mrs. Lyons. He was suffering from
a recurrence of encephalitis which had first attacked him
two years before. Though encephalitis is a viral disease
which sometimes can be cured, there are times when, apparently cured, it simply hides out in remission and
emerges in full force—a chronic disease now, insidious and
irreversible—as much as ten years later. Mr. Beale's disease had begun characteristically, with fever and headache and nausea, numbness in one leg, and double vision
(called diplopia). He was admitted to the hospital, treated,
and dismissed three weeks later. Considering himself
cured, he had resumed work (as an English professor at a
large midwestern university), but his energy had never
returned and the sexual impotence which had come upon
him several months before his illness had never reversed
itself. For nine months he'd suffered a gradually increasing lethargy, pains in his back, shoulders, and hips, constant distraction, and lapses in memory which grew more
and more embarrassing and demoralizing. Twice he was
admitted to hospitals, twice dismissed as "psychiatric."
Said one psychologist, whose report was in his files: "Mr.
Beale is a depressed man who is concerned about what he
perceives as his failing powers, particularly sexual, in the
context of more inclusive fears of personal inadequacies.
. . . It can be said that organic interference is not suggested." Psychiatric or not, within a year he was in-

capacitated. His memory loss, both short- and long-term, was definite and infuriating, causing tension and anger—going both ways—with everyone he knew. His two youngest children, whose names he no longer remembered, refused to eat while he was at the table. But like George Tinker's, his illness wasn't "real" until seizures confirmed it. Ten days ago, one day before his admission here, he'd called his wife's name from the couch where he now spent most of his time, then rolled onto the floor in a generalized convulsion. When she found him, she called an ambulance and—his "depression" now validated—he was admitted through the emergency ward.

Although his diagnosis was obvious, Beale was presented at Neurology Conference because the doctors wanted students and interns to have a look at his disease, which is relatively rare, and also because they wanted to determine whether a shunt (like so much neurological dysfunction, encephalitis can cause hydrocephalus) might help to relieve some of his acute symptoms. Before he was brought into the room, we heard from the neurology resident in charge of his case and a psychiatrist who'd had several sessions with both Beale and his wife. The first report was medicalese ("Examination on admission revealed a blue-eyed, one-hundred-eighty-three-pound, seventy-four-inch-tall, well-muscled, left-handed male with BPs in the one-sixteen-over-eighty range. . . . All phases of gait normal . . . deep tendon reflexes present . . . no palmomentals, Hoffmann's, jaw, snout, or Chvostek"), but the second offered another trip into the mind-brain dilemma that neurosurgeons try so hard to ignore. Beale's wife, it seemed, had noticed "personality changes" more than a year before his illness had begun. Heretofore conservative, an avowed academic, he had shocked her then when he began to talk of giving up his teaching position and devoting himself to poetry. At the same time, he became petulant and irritable, disorganized in his teaching, short-tempered with his children. In retrospect, said Mrs. Beale, it seemed that she had watched his attention span grow shorter day by day. Sex had died between them several months later, and a month after that he had confessed he was having an affair with one of his students. Two months later, his first "physical" symptoms appeared.

What was fascinating about the psychiatric material was not its substance (in all likelihood, the histories of most encephalitics would reveal similar tales) but its peculiar threat, the sense that it could destroy the meager clarity one had managed concerning Beale's disease. Did these symptoms mean that his neurochemical changes had caused his psychological problems, or had his chemistry proceeded from his psychology? Had his "mind" affected his "brain" or his "brain" his "mind"? If encephalitis is a virus infection, is one free to separate it from behavioral influence (locating it, perhaps, in that linguistic region of one's brain)? If so, what makes a brain susceptible to virus? If encephalitis caused changes in Beale's neurochemistry, could we not say that his love affair caused chemical changes too? Did George Tinker's brain-damaged son have something to do with the appearance of his brain tumor, or did the genetic inclination which produced his son's brain damage point him in the direction of meningioma, or were they completely unrelated? Such questions were always in circulation around neurological disease. For the purposes of treatment, they were ignored, but when they surfaced, they could quickly become obsessions. No one could ignore the paradox, but no one could solve it either, because at its root the neurology-psychology "problem" isn't scientific but linguistic. As Hughlings Jackson observed in 1878, the confusion is a function of how the problem is approached rather than of the manner in which the mind and brain are related:

> The doctrine I hold is: first, that states of
> consciousness (or, synonymously, states of
> mind) are utterly different from nervous
> states; second, that the two things occur
> together—that for every mental state there is
> a correlative nervous state; third, that
> although the two things occur in parallelism,
> there is no interference of one with the other.
> This may be called the doctrine of
> concomitance. . . . It seems to me that [this
> doctrine] is, at any rate, convenient in the
> study of nervous diseases. . . . I do not try to
> show what is the nature of the relation
> between mental and nervous states.

What this means is that "mind" and "brain" are concepts, and like most concepts they need not be related in
terms of cause and effect. Since the words "brain" and
"mind" do not exist in the same grammatical context, explaining events in one in terms of events in the other is no
more reasonable, or profitable, than explaining events in
both in terms of contemporary politics, or the redness of
an apple in terms of its taste. "The full exposition of an
object in nature (such as light)," writes Henry Edelheit in
an article on Jackson, "may require two hypotheses, each
so constructed that neither one can be expressed in terms
of the other." In effect, those who explain "brain" in terms
of "mind," or vice versa, are committing a philosophical or
grammatical error, and proof of the error will always be
found in the endless causality it generates; for example, if
Mr. Beale's love affair "caused" his encephalitis, what
brought about his love affair? And what brought about
what brought it about? Eventually, such arguments must
lead to postulation of First Cause (theology) or reevalua-
tion of the language that brought about the problem (posi-
tivism or linguistics). As Brockman put it once, "The brain-
mind problem may be interesting on a physiological or

pharmacological level, but no matter how you stretch your terms, you can't define a physical entity in terms of a nonphysical one."

The irony was that you could know all this, and agree with it, but retain your "incorrect" obsessions just the same. Surgeons could deal with the disease concretely (once seizures begin, the need to control them supersedes the need to understand them), and philosophers could deal with it abstractly, but if you were neither, if you were merely observing brain damage from a nonprofessional point of view, the obsessions with cause and effect or mind and matter could descend upon you like the plague. No matter how I disciplined myself, I could not suppress curiosity about Beale's love affair, the neurochemical changes it had induced and those which had made it possible.

Sometimes it seemed to me that the questions themselves were a kind of symptom, a function of brain damage in their own right, which had no more chance of being cured by "understanding" or "insight" than Beale's encephalitis did of being reversed by an understanding of his neurochemistry. But sometimes too my curiosity seemed correct and inevitable. The relation between brain and mind, after all, is the relation between material and immaterial, that which is visible and that which is not, that which is formed and that which is formless, and those relationships are explored by all human beings, consciously or unconsciously, throughout their lives. Who are not concerned with their own death, or the fragile line between life and death? To say of such questions, as Jackson did, that language cannot contain them, is not to say that they do not exist, but rather that their proper context is belief and intuition rather than language or analytic thought, religion rather than what we normally think of as scientific investigation. Mind-brain questions are asked throughout the Old and New Testaments, the Buddhist sutras, throughout Hindu mythology. "When you make the two one," Jesus said, "and when you make the inner as the outer and the outer as the inner and the above as the below ... then you shall enter [the Kingdom]." And the Buddhist text echoes him precisely: "Form is emptiness, and emptiness is form. Emptiness is not different from form, form is not different from emptiness." Mystical statements remind us that language is not reality, that Truth is always beyond our conceptual grasp. And the relationship of what we call "mind" to what we call "brain" is as supreme and ineffable as any truth that governs our existence. By breaking down the neat distinctions between psychology and neurology, people like Philip Beale could remind you of that ineffability and make you realize that mystics, after all, are no great fools in matters we call "scientific."

The resident in charge of Beale was an Argentinian named Ricardo, who had trained in London before coming here to work with Clarke. He was a large, humorless man with dark, oil-slick hair, cut short and combed in 1950s style. His information was inexhaustible and his presentation so monotonic and unfaltering that it seemed to come from a tape recorder. Unlike Lamar, he was secure in his position and fortunately so, because Mr. Beale was a bit more complicated than Mrs. Lyons. Like many chronic encephalitics, and people like Arthur Rodgers, Beale was emotionally labile, alternately belligerent, tearful, and ingratiating. As the history had noted, he was indeed well-muscled; he looked as if he had done some weightlifting in his youth and kept in shape until not so long ago. His eyes were penetrating and paranoid, hard to take for more than a few seconds. He seemed never far from the suspicion that we had caused his illness. What the history had not noted was that, while he had the appearance of a human being, he lacked something vital that might have made that appearance convincing. He seemed a collection of features waiting for unity, less a man than an approximation of one. It seemed he had just enough brain function to know that his own was insufficient.

During the interview, Ricardo looked at the audience and Beale stared at his hands, which he kept folded in his lap like a mischievous child pretending to be obedient. Questions and answers were quick and arrhythmical, as if both were reading from a script they did not completely understand.

RICARDO: Mr. Beale, I wonder if you would tell us why you're here.

BEALE: Why I'm here? My trouble seems to be a loss of memory. I meet someone this afternoon, see them tomorrow, it's gone.

RICARDO: Have you seen me before, sir?

BEALE: You seem familiar, but . . . no, I don't think so.

RICARDO: You don't remember our conversation this morning?

BEALE (with enthusiasm): Nope! I'm sorry, but . . .

At this point, Beale began to cry, leaning forward and shielding his eyes with his hand. When Ricardo touched his shoulder to comfort him, he screamed, "Watch it! Watch out!," then broke into a smile. "See you later, alligator!" he cried. "After a while, crocodile!"

Ricardo turned to the audience. "According to most sources on encephalitis, emotional lability of this type is more or less common in this sort of case." He turned to Beale again. "How did your illness begin, sir?"

"I'm vague about my own history. I think it was encephalitis. Anyhow, certainly, it was something in the system up here." Beale pointed to his head and, in a remarkable gesture, tapped his fingers on his skull as if playing the piano.

Ricardo asked a number of questions about his past— place of birth, family, education—and what Beale could answer was almost more interesting than what he couldn't. Why should he recall his first and second children's names but not his third and fourth? Why did he remember the name of his high school but not the name of his college? (One of the residents suggested that "See you later, alligator!" might have been popular when Beale was in high school, and that the part of the brain in which these memories resided had not been touched by the illness.)

RICARDO: Could you tell me what I do here, Mr. Beale?

BEALE: Kind of a personnel worker, aren't you? (He looked out the window, sobbing momentarily.) Now I'm trying to have an association come to my mind. You're working with people in roles and relations. Is that it?

RICARDO: Close to it. And what service are you on here at the hospital?

BEALE: Neurology?

RICARDO: Right. Why?

BEALE: I seem to have (he played the piano on his head again) a malfunction of the nervous system.

RICARDO: Do you know what that malfunction is?

BEALE: This has been complex for me. It involves memory and systems of orientation.

RICARDO: Were you here last night?

BEALE: Not that I recall. I was here. Yes, I was here.

When Ricardo finished, a sigh of relief ran through the room. Dreadful as it was, Beale's condition was not so extreme that one could avoid a touch of communion with him, and communion with encephalitis is as vivid a meeting with death as living persons are likely to endure.

Ricardo asked Clarke if he had seen enough and Clarke said no, he hadn't. "If Mr. Beale will bear with us, I would like you to test him on the definitions, so we can form a clearer picture of his deficit."

Beale nodded that he didn't mind (like Mrs. Lyons, he seemed to be enjoying himself), and Ricardo leafed through his notebook until he found the page he wanted —the standard definitions that neurologists employ to objectify confusion.

RICARDO: Would you tell me what these words mean to you, sir?

BEALE: Certainly!

RICARDO: Swellheaded?

BEALE: Sorry, I never heard of it. Could mean good, very good.

RICARDO: Conceited?

BEALE: That could mean expansion of the fluid areas, excess of flowing blood.

RICARDO: Tightfisted?

BEALE: Restricted. Does not open up for alterations of changing roles, specific content of statements.

RICARDO: What do we mean when we say, "When in Rome, do as the Romans do"?

BEALE: That refers to the Rome which includes the mass building of concrete homes and offices. Also could mean on the metaphysical side the Rome which has certain kinds of means the way people live, means of roles in society.

RICARDO: "Birds of a feather flock together"?

BEALE: This is one band of people who share certain kinds of meanings. On the other hand, people who share the same kinds of biophysical systems, using symbols, meanings, and so forth.

RICARDO: "Don't count your chickens before they hatch"?

BEALE: That means don't have claims for certain kinds of activities which are not existing in the social system.

After eighteen or twenty of these exchanges—each of which grew more convoluted as Beale, aware of his mistakes, tried to cover them up and so confused himself even more—Clarke called Ricardo off and mercifully (more for us, I think, than him) permitted Beale to return to his room.

Several moments of silence ensued before Brockman summed it up. "Not a chance," he said. "Forget it. We'll put in a shunt, but nothing's gonna help him now."

Several of the younger people ventured questions, but

no one offered much in response. Gloom as dark as any I
saw while at the hospital had settled on the room, a sudden
attack of that particular dread which physicians like to
think they've mastered through habituation. Clarke said,
"After his surgery, we'll send him over to the V.A. Thank
God he was in the army. He'll probably be there the rest
of his life."

Another meeting followed Neurology Conference, evening rounds followed that, and before rounds Brockman
saw several patients, one of whom, a former policeman,
had a bullet lodged in his head. The Boss would not leave
the hospital until just after nine in the evening on a day
that had begun—with his morning run—at 6:00 A.M.

The next meeting, called Rehab Rounds, was a gathering from the neurosurgery ward—nurses, social workers,
physical therapists, interns, and residents—to discuss patients currently on the floor. The problems here were mechanical and social: efforts to get Mr. Paget into a nursing
home, secure Tony Kirtz's insurance payments, arrange
with Mrs. Simpson's daughter to care for her when she
was sent home, readjust Mr. Maxwell's steroids in preparation for his surgery next week, and deal with the problem of Edwin Hawkesbury, the Haitian gentleman whose
mistress and wife—the latter claiming that the former
caused his tumor with a voodoo spell—had been screaming
at each other in the hall outside his room.

Brockman had sent down to the cafeteria for another
cup of coffee, smoked a few more cigarettes, taken another
peek at Marvin Welsh (now in the I.C.U.). If he was tiring,
he didn't show it. As usual, he seemed to feed on his activity, increase energy by expending it. He was relaxed here,
slightly paternal, more gentle and less aggressive than
anywhere else in the hospital. "You cut your hair," he said
to one of the nurses. "Looks good. Makes your eyes look
bigger."

When one of his patients—operated on a week before—
was described as "deteriorating," and one of the interns
observed that he was "no worse than before surgery,"
Brockman reprimanded him. "Like hell he isn't. Don't try
to make me feel good. You win some and you lose some.
Come on. We don't need to play games with each other."

There was a discussion about a new patient, a man with
a disk high in his spine that had prevented him from moving his neck for fifteen years; then a debate about a woman
whose seizures involved her whole face: were they prop-
erly to be called tics? If so, why were they so erratic?

"Hell," said the Boss. "She's just got a big sewer in her
head."

"Will she go home soon?" asked David.

"Yeah, why not?" he said. "She'll stroke eventually, but
there's nothing we can do about it."

As for Andy March, when Bryan described him as "withdrawing," Brockman said, "You mean he's getting ready
to die, don't you?"

Benny Richmond took out an index card and wrote a
note to himself. "I'll talk to his wife," he said, "and see if
she'll donate his eyes and kidneys."

When the nurses and social workers left, patients were
brought in. Those Brockman saw at this time were usually
special cases or emergencies who couldn't wait for regular
appointments or, like the policeman and the first patient
tonight, seekers of second opinion. The latter was a forty-
two-year-old electrician named Howard Judson, a tall, im-
pressive man of very few words, who had discovered three
weeks before (after a seizure) that he had an advanced
glioma. His first neurosurgeon had performed a biopsy to
get a piece of the tumor, then told him he would live maybe
fifteen months if he had surgery; nine at most—with disin-
tegrating language and memory—if he didn't. After
studying his angiogram, his CAT-scan, and the biopsy report, Brockman concurred. "That's a tumor that grows

very fast. We might be able to take a lot of it, but most of what we'd get would be back in six weeks."

Judson took it without flinching and stood up to leave without another question.

"Isn't there anything else you'd like to know?" Brockman said.

"No," he said. "I've got it all." (A week later, Brockman was informed by Judson's wife that after their meeting Howard had spent a week arranging his affairs, held a small going-away party with several intimate friends, and then killed himself with sleeping pills.)

The cop's name was Clifford Sachs. He was a square-jawed, frightened forty-year-old with a deep suntan (living in Arizona on his disability pension), prematurely gray hair, the most fascinating angiogram I ever saw, and a beautiful wife who could not tolerate his being the center of attention.

"Guess who's the patient!" she cried, as they sat down.

"Not you, that's for sure," Brockman said. "No patient would say such a thing."

Shot by a holdup man, Sachs had remained conscious, feeling no pain, until the ambulance arrived, then lapsed into an eight-day coma. When he awoke he was blind in his left eye, numb on the left side of his face, and quite miraculously free of other neurological deficit. His condition today—five years later—was the same. The reason for his visit was concern expressed by another neurosurgeon, himself a former student of Brockman's, that the bullet was pressing on his optic nerve and thus doing further damage. Angiography had been scheduled for tomorrow, surgery three days later.

"Somebody suggested we oughta talk to you," said Sachs's wife, "before we went ahead with it."

They had brought his old angiogram, and Benny mounted it on the screen. White against the dark background, the bullet shone like a defect in the negative, a silver streak that turned the X-ray into a painting. Benny whistled, and Brockman said, "Well, I guess we aren't gonna call you a liar, are we?"

Since he carried no instruments himself, he took Benny's ophthalmoscope and leaned over Sachs to have a look at his eye. Squinting, moving the scope in a circle, he muttered to himself, "Dead as Clancy's nuts. Come here, Benny. Did you ever see absolute optic atrophy?"

While Benny and the other residents looked through the scope and so monopolized Sachs's attention, the Boss leaned back and explored eye contact with the wife. I knew he had vowed to abstain with patients' wives, but since neither showed an inclination to retreat, I thought the vow might be erased just then on the examination table. Fortunately, Sachs's examination came to an end and, although the rest of the interview was directed to her and appeared to be fired by their exchange, priorities were readjusted. Say that once again he was rescued by his ability to forget. That and the rage he felt at the surgeon who had recommended Sachs's operation.

"Angiography!" he cried. "Can you believe it, Benny? And surgery, for Christ's sake! That's the goddamnedest misuse of medical knowledge I ever heard. I'm ashamed of him. We trained him to be a surgeon, not a businessman. Look here," he said, turning to Sachs. "That optic nerve is deader than shit. Nothing's gonna bring it back. And your seventh nerve is finished too. Working on your face is not gonna bring back your sensation. You're awful goddamn lucky to be alive. Take what you've got and don't try for more. The bullet is lodged in bone. It's never gonna move. There's no need for another angiogram, and God knows there's no justification for surgery. Wait till I get hold of that sonofabitch."

Sachs was astonished. "Nothing to worry about? Are you sure?"

"Absolutely. You'll never have that eye and you'll never

have sensation in your face, but you don't have to restrict your activities."

"I can play tennis?"

"I told you—play anything you want."

Brockman stood up, terminating the interview, but Sachs and his wife were too stunned to move. One question followed another: What if he bumped his head? What about lying in the sun? What about smoking and drinking and driving? In each case, the Boss assured him that he had nothing to worry about.

Finally, they stood up to leave, thanking him as if he had saved Sachs's life (which he may well have done).

"How much do we owe you?"

"Nothing. I don't charge policemen. I'm an honorary police surgeon myself, you know?"

Sachs went out first, but the woman turned back at the door, the barest smile acknowledging, it seemed to me, what had passed between them before. "And you're absolutely sure that nothing's going to move?"

Brockman, smiling himself, returned the favor. "No, sweetheart, not unless you move it for him."

Throughout rounds and for two days after that, he railed at the surgeon who had treated Sachs. "That fucker's gotten too big. Lost his clinical judgment. When you get that way, you never get enough cases. Last year he scared a lady to death. She'd had a subarachnoid hemorrhage thirteen years before, and he told her she had a time bomb in her head. Shit, statistics show that only one percent a year rebleed. And these days, if we even suspect they might, we treat them with hypotensive drugs. Time bomb, my ass. And you know what he'll say when I point it out? 'Jim's getting old.' If anything, he'll be angry at me."

Slapping his fist against his palm, he turned to Benny as they started toward the hall for rounds. "If there's anything a surgeon's got to watch out for, it's that: surgical ego, busywork. Some of these fuckers get so hooked on the O.R. they lose sight of their patients altogether. Remember what I say, Benny. There's nothing worse can happen to a surgeon than that sort of compulsive need to work."

Since residents did most of the dirty work and most decisions were made during Rehab Rounds, evening rounds were less a practical than a symbolic exercise, a meeting with patients and families that offered everyone, including Brockman, a chance for recapitulation. For doctors, rounds were brief resumptions of human contact in a situation that could become grotesquely impersonal, a chance to find out if one was a healer or just a technician. Some surgeons make rounds at 6:00 A.M. in order to avoid families, but Brockman gave the families as much as the patients, realizing that most of the time they had it worse. Patients at least could focus on their disease, but families had nothing to do but stand around and wait. If what he had to say was difficult ("Listen, his cells are crazy-looking; I don't know what to make of them"), he would take them to the nurses' station, but if it wasn't, he would keep them in the room during the examination.

Sometimes the hall was a mob scene during rounds. Patients with large families could turn the Visitors' Lounge into a cocktail party, spreading pizza or delicatessen on the tables, stacks of magazines and newspapers, Scrabble boards, beer cans, overnight bags crammed with anything they thought the patient might require. Every night they waited beside the patients with questions, complaints, fears, carefully written lists so Brockman wouldn't leave before they'd mentioned everything: new sensation in a plegic limb, night sweats, inexplicable pain. He came around with his entourage, sometimes four or five residents and a couple of interns and nurses, and while he was there, even for a few minutes after he left, everything was fine. Patients would tell you that if he said, "How're you

doing?" and you said, "Not so good," you felt better for
having said it. Sometimes five minutes could pass before
you'd realize nothing had changed.

We waded through the crowd that had collected around
the nurses' station ("Dr. Brockman? Have you seen the
X-rays yet? Can we go home this weekend?") and began
rounds as usual in I.C.U. Marvin Welsh was in the first
bed, just to the left of the door, wired up like a Rube
Goldberg machine, still zonked on his anesthesia. Brockman leaned down and hollered in his ear.

"Hi, Marvin! I'm Dr. Brockman! Remember me?"

"Ummmm."

"How you doin', kid?"

"Ummmm."

"That's great, really great, kid. Can you squeeze my
hand? Ah, wonderful, wonderful. Listen, Marvin, you're
doing fine! The operation went well. Everything's okay!
Keep it up!"

Next was Penny DeCarlo, the young woman who had
thrown herself in front of a bus. She was conscious, but
barely, breathing through an oxygen mask, one leg in
traction and another in a foam-rubber cast. She had frac-
tured her skull, six ribs, her femur, and her pelvis, but she
would survive, as a paraplegic, go home six months later
after long rehabilitation training. Since she would be
treated under the spinal-cord grant, Sarah Pincus, coordinator of that program, was in charge of her case. Sarah
had already interviewed Penny's family and thus developed a superficial psychological profile to rationalize the
suicide attempt, which seemed to have grown out of tension in her marriage. Penny and her husband, a lawyer,
had been fighting since they'd met, five years before, and
after the last battle she'd gone out "for a walk" and waited
for the bus. When she regained consciousness, she'd found
her husband standing beside her bed. Her first words

formed the basis of Sarah's profile: "Is it all right now if I don't have children?"

After Penny there was Irving Levy, who had come in with a tumor adjacent to his language region. Although he was sixty-eight and had terrible prospects from every point of view, Brockman had taken a shot at the tumor because attendant to it there had been seizures and parkinsonian symptoms (tremors and tics and right-side palsy). Once inside, however, he'd found the tumor harder and more widespread than he had expected, so he had taken only a fraction. Now, Levy was sitting up in a chair with his two daughters beside him, but he couldn't talk or, as far as anyone could tell, understand what was said to him. At his age, there wasn't much hope he would ever get better.

"Hi, Irving. You gonna talk to me today?"

"Hasn't said a word," whispered one of the daughters.

"Has he recognized you?"

"Not that we can see."

"Irving! Raise your leg!

Miraculously, Irving's foot shot up in the air until his leg was parallel to the floor. It was the first time since surgery that he'd obeyed a command. But then no one could get him to put his leg down. They asked him politely, commanded him, tapped his foot, and struck him a soft karate chop on the instep, but the foot stayed where it was. Finally one of the residents lowered it forcefully, gripping it behind the knee.

Brockman turned to the daughter. "We'll increase his steroids and hope for the best. If he's not better by next week, he won't get better at all." With a younger patient, he might have operated again, but at Irving Levy's age there wasn't much sense in that. Steroids were all he had to offer.

There were thirty patients to see that evening, twelve

postop (three long-term, receiving radiation therapy), seven preop, four diagnostic, three in the rehabilitation wing, two in pediatrics, two in neurology (their surgical prospects still undetermined). At least twenty of these patients had families who required explanation, advice, prognosis, or consolation. One husband was furious that the Boss wanted Kellogg, rather than himself, to do his wife's aneurysm; another wanted to know what his wife could do when she came home from the hospital ("Anything but drive"). A wife was panicked because she had discovered "a soft spot" on her husband's skull. And finally, Mrs. March, having sat with her husband through eighteen days of coma, inquired obliquely as to the possibilities of euthanasia.

"If he's in pain . . . isn't there something . . . some way . . . do you think I'm wrong to ask?"

Obviously it wasn't the first time Brockman had heard such a question, but his position precluded a simple answer. If he complied with her wish, he was subject to criminal prosecution or a lawsuit for malpractice, but if he denied it, he was denying what he knew to be the only intelligent course of action. "All I can do," he said, "is take him off the support systems, like we've already done. And of course increase his pain medication, which, as you know . . . well, we'll see what happens."

He was about to explain to her that increasing the medication would make her husband more susceptible to infection, but once again the specter of malpractice loomed, and he thought better of it.

"Do you think she understood?" he asked Benny when we came out of the room.

"No," Benny said.

Food smells circulated. Swiss steak or flounder for dinner tonight, mashed potatoes, carrots and peas, Jell-O or ice cream. As usual, television was clamorous, ubiquitous, no small comic relief. Sets, as I mentioned earlier, were pushed aside but seldom turned off when he came in, and many meetings were accompanied by the sound track. Sometimes you would look around and see the residents and nurses, everyone but the Boss and the patient, riveted on the screen. Another thing you could do was eat. Almost every bed had a store of cookies, candy, and homemade cakes nearby, and patients—many of whom had no appetite—were thrilled if you'd accept them. It got around quickly which beds had the best selection, and as we approached that room on rounds, a couple of the residents and one of the interns could be seen to quicken their pace. They'd take a cookie as they came in, help themselves during the interview (if the Boss wasn't looking), and, if the fare was especially good, fill their pockets for the road. Stories were told of residents who had grown obese during service here, but I think they were apocryphal: their hours were so ridiculous and their meals so irregular that most were thin as rails.

"Who remembers inorganic chemistry?" said Brockman as we left Andy March's room. "My grandson wants to build a volcano." We discussed the problem in the hall (the residents could not agree, and Brockman had no memory of chemistry at all) until we were interrupted by the father of a boy who had been operated on by Ken Beck for a pituitary tumor: was it possible to say whether the female characteristics which had been caused in his son by the tumor would be reversed by surgery?

Brockman smoked without interruption during rounds, often disappearing into the bathroom to flick a butt toward the toilet. As in the operating room, teaching was constant: "Flex your muscles, Benny! Goddamn it, sometimes I think you're too nice to be a neurosurgeon!" "Jesus, are you guys serious? Why don't you look at the patient for a change? What about her night sweats? What are you doing here if you're gonna be sleeping all the time?"

Treatment was not always democratic. Brockman had

favorites among his patients, as well as an instinct for which would be helped and which hurt by too much attention. Young, good-looking females could keep him in their rooms for ten or fifteen minutes with questions which, with another patient, he would have answered over his shoulder as he hurried toward the door. He always spent a good deal of time with patients about to be released after surgery, preparing them as best he could for the return to real life. And elderly Jewish matriarchs could keep him as long as they wanted.

Outside each room, Benny read from his index cards, briefing the Boss on the patient he was about to see. "This is the forty-nine-year-old woman with the parasagittal meninge." "This is the Spanish lady with sensory loss at T-three." "This is the sixty-seven-year-old man with the third-grade astrocytoma." If patients were new, admitted during the day or over the weekend, briefing was more detailed. "This is a fifty-seven-year-old white man who presented with loss of consciousness, headaches, one seizure, and confusion. The CAT-scan shows pickup in the left temporal lobe." Brockman took in just enough to revive his memory ("That was the right hemisphere, wasn't it?") or, if the patient was new, to prepare himself for the meeting, and then, with a flourish nearly regal, marched into the room with his entourage behind him. "Hi! I'm Dr. Brockman!"

From Andy March we went to Clemencia ("How are you tonight, Clemencia?" "Sorry, doctor, I'm not at liberty to say") and her roommate, Ethel Peterson, who was aphasic and terminal.

"How are you tonight, Ethel?"

"How are you, doctor?"

"I'm fine, thanks, how are you?"

"How are you, doctor?"

"Great! What about you?"

"How are you, doctor?"

The next room was better news. Mrs. Kraus, who had been plegic on her left side, had some of her shoulder back. Brockman was thrilled. "Didn't I say you'd be okay? Didn't I give you my word?"

"Does this mean I'll be a human being again?"

"Hell, Betty, you're a human being now. Isn't she, fellas?"

She was a large, jolly woman, one of his Jewish matriarchs, and she treated him with less respect than almost any other patient, commanding him now. "Sit down. I've got some complaints."

"No time, no time. I've heard enough of your complaints."

"I said, sit down! I've got a right to complain. I'm a Jewish woman!"

In Room 934, things were as I'd left them. Arthur Rodgers and Raymond Dreyer were watching television, and Mr. Sedgwick and Dr. Chardan were still arguing. They asked Brockman whether in his opinion Sedgwick's operation had been a waste of time.

"No," the Boss replied. "You'd a been dead in six months if you hadn't had it."

"So what?" Sedgwick said.

Brockman turned away. "That's for you to say, not me."

In the next-to-last room was Mr. Adelman, a big name in local politics, who had come in three days before with what had turned out to be a blood clot on the outside of his brain. It had been drained in a fairly uncomplicated procedure, and soon he would go home. This was the only patient I ever heard the Boss single out for special attention. "Listen, you guys, be good to this guy. If anyone's gonna get us another CAT-scan, it's him."

At eight forty-five we were in a room that faced Brockman's apartment house across the street. Leaning over the patient, he glanced out the window and said to no one in particular, "Hey, my wife's home from work!" Ten minutes later, he would leave and walk across the street, where, as usual, he'd have two Scotches and a light dinner, watch the evening news on television, and put himself to sleep by listening to the all-news station through an earphone on the radio beside his bed. ("My invention," he said proudly. "I defy anyone to stay awake through the basketball scores.")

The last patient was Edna McCarthy, a seventy-year-old terminal (metastasized) cancer patient who had been an accomplished professional painter before her illness. As Brockman left her room, her son followed him into the hall, explaining that Mrs. McCarthy wanted to know, for the purposes of her work, how long she could expect to live.

"Tell her she won't be here in a year, but she might in six months."

9

The Music Lessons

Behold your body—
A painted puppet, a toy,
Jointed and sick and full of false imaginings,
A shadow that shifts and fades.

—Buddha Sakyamuni

Five days later, Charlie White returned. By now his view of surgery as adventure had given way to something darker and a bit less heroic, but it was a sweet late-April afternoon and, as he got off the bus, breezes from the river rekindled the crazy excitement he'd felt just after his seizure, the sense that he was graced somehow by his predicament, that surgery would be the quintessential moment of his life.

It was now more than four weeks since his tumor had announced itself, and it seemed to him that nothing in his life had escaped its influence. He was different with friends, impatient with small talk and slightly pontificating, offering advice like an old soldier back from the war. Most of the friendships he'd sustained throughout his twenties struck him now as superficial. He had given up an apartment he never liked, quit a job that had always seemed beneath him. The life he'd live when he recovered had become an endless source of fantasy.

The book he had wanted to write on neurosurgery had now become a novel. In his overnight bag he carried writing materials, the tape recorder with which, with Roberta's help, he hoped to collect his first words on coming out of anesthesia, and (groundwork for the novel) several books about the brain. He knew he'd be too frightened to read before surgery, but it seemed to him that afterward, if he survived, reading about the brain would be the perfect way to pass the time. No way to know that reading, for the next three weeks, would be impossible. That mostly he'd want to lie in bed and look at the ceiling and think about the mess beneath his bandage. That although his mind would clear within four days after surgery, reading would seem like a "risk," a disturbance of the equilibrium in the region around his wound. In fact, he would read nothing while at the hospital except the front page of one morning paper, five days after surgery, and when he developed a headache later that afternoon, he would be sure that reading had brought it on. ("It's too soon for mental exertion.") Neurosurgery may not involve the mind, but sooner or later, usually sooner, the connection will be drawn between the incision and thoughts about it.

Charlie was issued a dressing gown and assigned to Room 928, a double. In the bed beside him was Timothy Jenkins, a ballet dancer from Florida who was two days postop after risky spinal-cord surgery (a tumor at the highest vertebra, the ultimate all-or-nothing shot for Brockman: perfect health if the operation succeeded; death or quadriplegia if it failed) that had left him absolutely cured. Besides their age—thirty-one—their idolatry of

Brockman, and their addiction to the Boston Red Sox, the two men, like George Tinker and several others on the ward, shared a conviction that their illnesses were part of a larger violence, almost a poltergeist that had drawn their lives into its vortex. On the night Charlie was first brought to the hospital, his mother and sister were mugged on a street near their home. Two days later, Roberta came on a knife fight and assisted in apprehending a man who had attacked an elderly woman. A few days after that, Charlie's ex-girl friend had a breast cancer diagnosed, and her breast was removed two days before he returned to the hospital. In Timothy's family, four people—his mother, two uncles, and a cousin—had died within a month of his admission here.

It wasn't unusual to hear stories like this on the ward, and very often they were used to explain the onset of tumors and hemorrhage. The need to explain, of course, was desperate here. Why on earth should these things happen in one head rather than another? I heard tumors laid to diet, magic, misbehavior, worry, or this kind of karmic vicissitude, and there was no way to argue with any of it. No one knows why meningiomas or gliomas form, and no one knows why some brains are prone to aneurysm or seizures. If you want to lay it on karma or sin or eating too much junk food, there's no one in the world who can disprove your theory.

During the next thirty-six hours, Charlie had a chest X-ray, an EKG, a urinalysis, tests for kidney and liver function, and a series of blood tests to determine, among other things, his coagulation profile. There was no time to be afraid. When he wasn't being examined, he was moving around the hospital, talking with Timothy and other patients, taking calls from friends, visiting with his mother and his sister. When there was free time, he took notes for the novel. Under such conditions it wasn't difficult to think of the hospital as a hotel. There was television at night and a couple of good-looking nurses, the sheets were clean, and the meals, if nothing special, were edible and ample. No shopping to do, no dishes to wash, nothing to take to the Laundromat, and the view from the room was beautiful. Thinking of surgery was like trying to imagine a movie you planned to see. He did not realize how pervasive his denial had become until Terry Schreiber stopped by to visit on the night before the operation.

Schreiber was chief of anesthesiology, the Boss's equivalent in his department, an expansive British eccentric with the body and bearing of an Olympic wrestler, a pro-Nixon political philosophy which led to endless arguments in the O.R., and (according to the nurses) a lust for the dollar which made it almost impossible for him to refuse a case. On the night he visited Charlie, he came straight from the O.R., where he'd done a brain tumor beginning at seven in the morning and a hip operation after a thirty-minute lunch break. When he left Charlie's room, he would have a quick dinner and go back to the O.R. for peripheral nerve surgery, which would last until six the following morning, when he would have breakfast and go to work on Charlie. When he finished with Charlie at about one forty-five the following afternoon, he would finally go home and to bed after thirty-one hours of almost uninterrupted work.

Meetings like this were standard on the night before surgery, an opportunity for the anesthesiologist to find out certain things he needed to know about his patient and perhaps—since induction of the anesthetic was in many cases the focus of presurgical terror—to undermine anxiety. In Charlie's case, unfortunately, denial at this point leaving nothing to undermine but itself, Schreiber's visit marked the beginning of the end. By the time he left, Charlie's terror was everywhere he turned.

After a series of standard questions—"All those teeth yours? Any loose or cracked teeth? Any conditions for which you see a physician regularly? Any serious illness in your past? TB? Polio? Rheumatic fever?"—Schreiber abandoned formality and, leaning over the bed with a diabolical grin, entered upon his peculiar technique for putting patients at their ease.

"Look here, sport, you're a very lucky man. I happen to be the best anesthesiologist in the world. But you should also know that I'm a black belt in karate. If you don't do what I say, I'll give you a chop"—he demonstrated on his own palm—"that will separate you from your head. Now listen to me closely. I'm serious. When you wake up tomorrow, you're gonna be fine. No aftereffects, I give you my word. But two things you've got to remember: don't cough and don't flail with your arms.* Got it? Don't cough and don't swing your arms. If you do, I'll leave the room, and you know what that means, don't you?"

"No," Charlie said. "What does it mean?"

Schreiber didn't answer the question at first but let it circulate while he watched Charlie with a smile that was almost tender. Rough as he sounded, most patients loved him because he played with them and forced them out of their fear. He took Charlie's hand in his, gripping him by the thumb. "It doesn't mean anything, because you'll do what I say. All you have to do is repeat it to yourself a couple of times tonight and tomorrow morning, and then you'll control it automatically."

After he left, the night nurse came with forms to be signed:

AUTHORIZATION FOR MEDICAL TREATMENT,
ADMINISTRATION OF ANESTHESIA
AND THE PERFORMANCE OF OPERATIONS
AND/OR PROCEDURES.

---

* Coughing would increase intracranial pressure, and arm movement would interfere with the I.V. and arterial lines installed during surgery.

I hereby authorize Dr. James Brockman to perform upon me the following medical treatment and/or procedures. . . . It has been explained to me that, during the course of the operation, unforeseen conditions may be revealed or encountered which necessitate surgical or other procedures in addition to or different from those contemplated. I therefore further request and authorize the above named surgeon or his designees to perform such additional surgical or other procedures as he or they deem necessary or desirable. . . . The nature and purpose of the operation and/or procedures, the necessity therefor, the possible alternative methods of treatment, the risks involved and the possibility of complication in the treatment of my condition have been fully explained to me and I understand the same. I recognize that the practice of surgery is not an exact science and I acknowledge that no guarantees or assurances have been made to me concerning the results of such procedures.

When the nurse went out, Charlie had several moments to ponder what he'd read. Then Brockman stopped by for evening rounds.

"You scared?"

"Yeah, I guess so, a little."

"Of what?"

"I don't know."

"Yes, you do. You're afraid you're gonna die."

"Well, sure, why not?"

"Don't be. We'll take care of you. We know what we're doing. Okay?"

"Yeah, okay."

"Anything you want to know?"

Charlie laughed. "I don't want to know anything. What do you want to know?"

Brockman took his hand. "We know what we need to know. We're all set. We'll get as much tumor as we can and hope we don't do you any damage. As long as you keep laughing, kid, you'll do all right."

Charlie closed his eyes and sighed. When he finally spoke, he seemed closer to tears than at any time since I'd met him. "Don't let it fool you, doc. I'm laughing on the outside. But I'm crying on the inside."

He tried to watch the ball game, talk sports with Timothy, but it was no use. His mother and Roberta had showed up during rounds, but they were worse off than he was, leaving the room every few minutes to have a cry in the hall. He felt terrible when they were there, worse when they went out. When visiting hours ended, there was a moment of relief, a sense that the fear was less unshared than shared, and even a brief resumption of the overview that made all of it seem instructive and heroic. Then the terror rose again, concrete views of surgery now: grotesque images of his head split open, the Boss's hands wrist deep inside his skull. Later he'd liken the fear to being swallowed by a whale.

"You okay?" Timothy said.

"No, I guess I'm not."

"Watch the ball game."

"I can't."

"Watch it anyway."

At nine they gave him a Valium—which as far as he could tell had no effect whatever—and a few minutes later, the priest stopped by to bless him. He requested a special blessing on his tumor, and after pulling the curtains around his bed to give them privacy, the priest obliged.

At nine thirty Benny came to shave his head. Charlie had been prepared for this trauma (every patient warned you about it; according to Benny, women and teenage boys often went to pieces at this point), but to his amazement, the sight of the clippers evoked nothing in him, and the feeling of his head, tiny without hair, rough "like sandpaper" on the surface, was nearly pleasant. Perhaps the Valium was helping after all. In any event, it seemed to him that the haircut—and the watch cap, which Benny presented first for his approval, then fitted on his head—marked the end of his fear, the end, in a sense, of his natural, ordinary life, and the entry into the netherworld of surgery. He said nothing now, shrugging his shoulders when Timothy asked him how he felt, but later he would remember this moment as his release, comparing it to the sensation one has when an airplane turns on the runway and accelerates for takeoff. "It was out of my hands, so I gave up worrying. Nothing to do but let it be. I felt absolutely calm."

Charlie slept soundly. No dreams that he recalled. When I came in the following morning, he said, "Whatever happens, man, it was meant to be. I've put my faith in the team downstairs and the Man upstairs."

But that statement was the beginning of a manic rap that would not stop until he went to sleep on the table. He had an idea for a television commercial (jotting it down in his notebook) to aid "the fight against crime"; several thoughts about the Red Sox pitching staff and an idea for a trade he thought could win them the pennant; an insight concerning hospital administration, to cut costs in the area of food preparation. He told Polish jokes and argued baseball with Timothy. His eyes were crazy-bright the way they'd been at his first meeting with Brockman, shifting as quickly as his mood. In turn he was stoical, joyous, avuncular, philosophical, platitudinous. Often he lectured himself as if no one else were in the room. "Whatever happens, man, it's got to be. This too shall pass. Stand tall, that's the main thing. Be proud of yourself when it's over." His eyes spread wide and his conversation ceased whenever someone entered the room. Just before they came for him, he motioned me close and whispered, "Don't let it fool you. I'm scared shitless."

There was much to do to get him ready. Just after he woke, a nurse plugged an I.V. into his right wrist to start him on steroids and decrease his intracranial pressure. Orally, he got Dilantin and phenobarbital for seizures, Nembutal for terror. This last—since sedatives affect the brain—was a concession they did not like to make around here. Older patients, their brains a bit too impressionable for Nembutal, got nothing but Benadryl before going downstairs.

The night nurse, on duty now until 8:00 A.M., was the best and toughest I had seen around the ward. She was a dark-haired, middle-aged woman with a Slavic accent, chiseled features, and eyes that told you she'd sent an awful lot of patients downstairs. She did things quickly but without haste, acknowledged anxiety without catering to it. Everything she said to Charlie was a command ("Give me your arm; take your Dilantin"), until she was done with him and about to move on to other patients. Then she allowed herself a smile and, pressing his hand, spoke what I'd remember as the most eloquent words I heard during my time at the hospital. "Good luck, Charlie. I know you'll make it 'cause you got spirit. See you tonight."

The attendant from the operating room—they call them runners—was a Puerto Rican who spoke almost no English and smelled of a potent after-shave lotion. He was kind and cheerful, a small, stocky fellow wearing gold-rimmed spectacles, but in this context it was difficult not to see him as an executioner. He carried a clipboard.

"Charles White?"

"Yes?"

"I'm from the operating room."

"Yeah?"

"Yeah."

Charlie leaned and gripped Timothy's hand, forcing a
smile. "See you later, old man." As his bed was wheeled
into the hall, he whispered, "Shitless, shitless," several
times in my direction, then turned back to Timothy at the
door. "Hey, Tim, don't forget to have them turn off my
television. Why should I pay for it if I can't use it?" And
then his bed moved down the hall, rolling toward the elevator.

When he reached the operating floor, he joined a line of
patients waiting for surgery, seven beds backed up from
the swinging doors like planes stacked for takeoff. Charlie
had forgotten me, though I was standing just behind him.
Maniacally, his voice obsessive and breathless, he repeated, "This is it," and crossed himself at least half a
dozen times. The space between us was vast now, the wall
around him thicker and more impenetrable as he drew
close to surgery. I watched him as if he were exotic, a
foreign creature whose mind and mood had almost nothing
in common with my own. He seemed outside of time, frozen in space like a photograph. Nothing about him was
ambiguous and nothing accessible.

By the time they took him in, the operating room was
ready. The scrub nurses, my old friend Millie Yates and
her assistant, Esther Woolf, had arrived at seven. Since
the night nurse, first, and then the porters, had cleaned
and prepared the room (as Millie and Esther would prepare
it for the team who would use it this afternoon), they
devoted themselves to the instruments and the equipment
for craniotomy. As usual, while they had the room to themselves, they danced and sang along with music on Esther's
transistor radio. They were two lovely women in their mid-
twenties, their energy and health (especially now, while
they danced around the room) a mockery of the work they
did. Both preferred the O.R. to the ward because, as
Esther put it, they didn't like sick people. "I don't know
what to say to them or how to touch them." Esther had

been at it for two years and Millie for four, working all the rooms, neuro and ortho, as they called them, and heart and general, and though they never stopped complaining or raging against the surgeons, they were skillful and resilient under a great deal of pressure. How else could they deal with the demands and idiosyncrasies of men like Brockman and Kellogg?

It was their job to clear the path for the surgeons, make certain everything was clean and sterile and available when needed, machines at hand but not underfoot, videotape in order, drill bits cleaned and sharpened, lights angled correctly. They were expected to anticipate instruments two or three steps ahead of the surgeons, so that when the Boss said, "Mosquito," and a resident said, "Bayonet," they would have both instantaneously and pass them correctly while preparing the next request, so that what Brockman called "the rhythm of surgery" was never interrupted. In some hospitals it was not unheard-of for nurses—if surgeons got to them—to walk out in the middle of an operation, but Osler was a prestige job; it paid too well and taught too much to permit such emotional responses. One was expected to contain anger and fatigue and understand the operation almost as well as the surgeon.

Of all the rooms they'd worked, both Millie and Esther and Lisa King, who joined them later, called neuro the most difficult and the most intense. In fact, there were some nurses who would not work this room at all. Besides the symbolic connotation of working on the brain and the much-publicized hysteria of neurosurgeons, there were practical aspects to consider, the fact that more instruments were required here than in other rooms, and the fear that Esther called the abiding obsession of those who worked in neurosurgery, the one that kept her awake at night, sometimes, even after she'd adapted to the room. "You can drop things on the heart, but not on the brain."

When José Rivera arrived at seven twenty, most of the machines were in place and the instruments laid out, rolled in blue towels, on the stand that straddled the operating table. Since the room was twenty-five years old, predating most of its technology, it was an electrical nightmare, and the greatest problem for Esther and Millie was keeping cords disentangled. Ten or fifteen electrical machines were used in an operation like this, each of them plugged to the wall, of course, and many connected in series, by other wires, to probes or pedals or sensors. If one included tubes like the catheters and the I.V. lines, there were thirty-four cords trailing across the floor, and many of these originated in machines that had to move during the course of surgery. Five lines came from the electrocardiogram and three from the anesthesia machine, and the electrocoagulation equipment, using foot pedals, required six lines of its own.

While Esther worked with the operating microscope (wheeling it out of a large closet, wrapping it in plastic, and securing the plastic with masking tape), Millie climbed on the stool that served the scrub table and busied herself with the instruments. Every morning she prepared 150 tools. No need here to furnish the list, but it included such wondrous items as a "joker elevator" and two "brain needles," a "Russian forceps," and a "long curved Kelly." In addition to these, bone wax was required (for sealing off holes drilled in the skull) and sutures and needles, five syringes (disposable; glass syringes are obsolete), drapes and towels, five different kinds of coagulant material, and endless packs of sponges, which before and after surgery were counted aloud, for legal purposes, to make sure none had been left inside the patient.

The first thing José did was mount Charlie's X-rays on a screen behind the operating table. Then he turned off Millie's radio. "All right, ladies. Enough fun and games. Time to get to work."

"Yes, papa," Esther said.

"What's the case?" Millie asked.

"Motor-strip meninge. Nothing special."

When Millie finished on the stand, she took the handles which were used to manipulate the huge, drum-shaped lamps that moved in tracks along the ceiling and inserted them in the sterilization machine that was built into the wall. Most instruments had been sterilized by the night nurse before he left, but these handles, which had been touched and therefore contaminated as they arranged the room, and would be touched by the surgeons while they worked, had to be sterilized again before the operation began.

At seven thirty, fifteen minutes after Charlie had come down to the floor, Esther went out to the hall for him. A moment later the big bed pushed through the door, made a sharp turn, backed up, moved sideways, forward, and sideways again, and finally came to a stop parallel to the operating table. Millie asked if he could lift himself and slide across. "Why not?" he said, and then, as if they had done him a favor, "Thank you very much."

By now his "calm" was frozen, his face white, and his mouth locked in a smile that seemed almost contorted. Many of his reactions were incongruous and disproportionate. He replied "Thank you" to almost anything said to him, and when José tapped his wrist softly in preparation for another I.V. line, he cried, "Ow!" as if the needle had already broken skin. They had removed his dressing gown and covered him with a sheet, buckled leather straps across his chest and thighs. In turn he looked terrified, helpless, innocent, and oblivious. Since the pace of the room had quickened, he was a still point in the midst of great activity. Now that Benny and Lisa had arrived, there were five people working on him, plugging him into machines, moving his legs, tilting the table, applying leads for the EKG to his chest and a blood-pressure strap to his arm.

They were ignoring him, and he was talking to himself. "This is it, baby. This is the real thing. Unbelievable! What a joke. A joke? Yeah, sure, but a real one, a real one."

Since the room was kept very cold—mostly for the surgeons, who could become uncomfortably warm during the course of an operation*—he was shivering badly, but he did not ask for a blanket.

"Are you cold?" Lisa said.

"Yeah, maybe I am."

"Want a blanket?"

"Maybe, yeah. Thank you very much."

"How's that?"

"Fine, fine, thanks very much."

"Can I do anything else for you?"

"Yes, get me out of here."

"Anything else?"

"Could you scratch my forehead?"

"There?"

"A bit to the left."

"There?"

"That's it. Thanks very much."

"How much do you weigh?" Benny said.

"Why do you ask?"

"We need to know. How much you weigh?"

"One-sixty. Why?"

"We need to know."†

Charlie caught a glimpse of me in the corner and broke out a grin. For a moment, to my amazement, he seemed almost happy. "Shitless, wow!" he whispered, and then, "If Marcus Welby comes through that door, I've had it. Anybody here seen *Coma?*"

"I did," Esther said. "I loved it."

---

* One famous neurosurgeon was said to have an air-conditioning unit built into his scrub suit.
† Several drugs administered during surgery are given in proportion to body weight.

"Not me," Benny said. "I thought they ruined it in the end."

"Who is Marcus Welby?" Lisa said.

"My God, woman," José said. "What country do you live in?"

Moods changed quickly here, as if winds blew them through the room. There was no way to avoid the knowledge of what was about to happen and no way, with the patient awake, to acknowledge it. The result was often this sort of mindless chatter, the sort of thing one might hear among people who've been drinking together or lying together on a beach.

All of it ceased abruptly with the arrival of Terry Schreiber. Theatrical though he was, he brought a sense of danger to the room, as though things were about to take a turn that no one could control.

"Good morning, ladies! Good morning, gentlemen. How are we today?"

Schreiber carried an attaché case and a clipboard, which he put down on the anesthesia stand. Turning to Charlie, he said, "How you doing, sport?"

"Okay, I guess."

"Remember what I told you last night?"

"Don't cough, right?"

"What else?"

"Don't swing my arms?"

"Right! Excellent!"

He broke open an I.V. kit and quickly found the vein he wanted in Charlie's wrist.

"You're gonna feel a little prick now, sport, but nothing bad. And then you're gonna sleep real sound. As a matter of fact, you're gonna have the sweetest sleep you ever knew. Ready?"

Charlie didn't answer. He was looking at the ceiling.

"Good night, sport. Remember now: no coughing!"

The first agent was sodium pentothal, administered

through the I.V. line. Having set up the line and connected it to a bottle overhead, Schreiber opened a syringe, filled it from a bottle, then injected it into the line.

"Good night, sport," he said again, and before half the syringe was empty Charlie's head had keeled to the right.

With his departure, the room veered and increased its velocity maybe fifteen times, like a satellite shifting orbit. No appearance to maintain now, no need to screen the violence. Benny removed Charlie's cap and with a purple marking pen—centering himself by putting his little finger on Charlie's nose and his thumb on the peak of his skull —drew a freehand line along the midline of his skull, then another from ear to ear, bisecting it. With the arrival of Schreiber's assistant, Carla Fredericks, there were seven people working in the room. While Schreiber administered nitrous oxide through a mask and finally halothane (the principal agent, which would drip through the I.V. line throughout the operation), Carla inserted in Charlie's mouth a long plastic tongue depressor with a light on the end of it, and then, aiming an eight-inch needle down his throat, gave him a shot of lidocaine to anesthetize his vocal cords and prevent them from going into spasm from the general anesthesia. Withdrawing the syringe, she clamped a fearsome-looking gadget called a bitelock over his tongue and turned on the central I.V. line so that pancuronium, the paralytic agent administered along with the halothane, would demobilize every muscle except the heart, protecting Charlie from bucking during surgery and moving his tumor around. A moment later, as Charlie was now incapable of breathing for himself, she turned on the respirator, and the black accordion device, hanging above the table, began the expansions and contractions which would continue throughout the operation.

While Carla worked, José painted Charlie's penis with brown Betadine solution and slid a greased catheter up the hole and into his urethra, taped plastic covers over his eyes, inserted a needle and then a catheter in the femoral artery in his right thigh (to track his blood pressure), installed a line in his left hand through which, if required, he'd be given blood, and yet another in his right foot, as a precautionary measure, in case one of the other lines blocked. Esther placed a copper plate under his buttocks to ground the electrocoagulation equipment. And Carla, when she was done with the I.V. lines, inserted a rectal thermometer (very important, this: the operation would affect the hypothalamic regions that control body temperature), which through an electrical circuit gave readouts directly on the anesthesia machine.

Benny had recently returned from Cuba, and Schreiber was angry that he'd gone. Why would anyone visit a communist country? "This is the best country in the world! Try living somewhere else! Then you'll appreciate it!"

"I brought you some cigars," Benny said.

"I don't want none of their cigars."

"Jesus Christ," Millie said. "This guy works for the C.I.A."

"Laugh at me, I don't care. I know what I'm talking about. You people don't know how good you've got it. You ought to live in Russia for a while. That would set you straight."

It was seven fifty. José and Benny checked the angiograms, then moved back to Charlie's head to adjust its angle. Position is crucial in neurosurgery, often one of the most important decisions a surgeon makes. Sometimes they put patients on their stomachs, sometimes (when they have to enter at the base of the head) in sitting positions, with their chins on their chests. Once they had Charlie right, they mounted his head on a black rubber cushion with a hole in the center that looked like a huge chocolate doughnut. Since his neck muscles were paralyzed, only gravity was required to keep his head in place.

"Just about here, right?" José said, indicating an area on the top of the skull.

"Yes," Benny said. "Its anterior point not much beyond here, and its posterior extension, I'd say, just about here."

Using the lines Benny had drawn as guides, they marked the flap on Charlie's skull: five tiny circles and then a pentagon connecting them. As Brockman had indicated in his first meeting with Charlie, the horseshoe shape began and ended on each side at his ear and peaked beyond the midline of his skull.

That was as far as they could go before scrubbing, so they retired to the washroom across the hall, where they went through the elaborate cleansing ritual prescribed for all who will touch a patient. In their absence I took a good look at Charlie, the last time for a while that I would see his face, perhaps the last time altogether that I'd see his identity intact. I tried to feel appropriate emotion like fear or sorrow, dread, or some sort of queasiness at a minimum, but all of it seemed sentimental and willful, as out of place in the O.R. as the music from Esther's radio. At that moment I wasn't completely sure whether Charlie was on the table or somewhere else, having left his body off for repairs.

Since Benny and José could touch nothing after scrubbing, Millie completed their outfits. Like the rest of us they already wore scrub suits and had now donned their masks (Benny wore two masks because he had a cold that day and his nose was dripping over the first), but a bit more equipment was required for surgeons than those who watched or attended them. When they returned to the room, hands held high and still dripping from the wash, Millie slipped surgical gowns over their necks and then, over the gowns, a "back protector," tying each at the waist. Gradually, they grew thick, like football players strapping on their pads. The second scrub shirt was a sleeveless affair, the sleeves

separate this time so that, if one brushed against something and became contaminated, a new sleeve could be
added and sterilization achieved without a great deal of
fuss. The final touch, and one of the ultimate images in
the surgical iconography, was the brown, skintight rubber gloves, which Millie removed from plastic bags and
(not without difficulty, since they fit so tightly) drew
over their fingers and wrists and sleeves. The rubber
made a squeaking sound, like crepe soles on linoleum
floors, and when the gloves were secured, they looked
like sick, discolored skin. Finally, José and Benny were
anonymous. Nothing showed but their eyes. Caps pulled
over their necks, waving their rubber fingers at the
room, they could have passed as creatures from another
planet. To complete the effect, Millie clamped Benny's
headlight on his forehead (as second resident, José
would not require one) and adjusted it, as he faced
Charlie's head, so that it shone on the flap he'd drawn
with his marking pen. It might have been a third, a luminous, eye protruding from his skull.

Quickly now, Benny built drapes around Charlie, clamp-
ing green paper sheeting material to the operating table
and the instrument stand so that nothing showed but the
flap. Once more he went over its lines with his marking
pen, and then with a needle etched the lines into the skin,
sending trickles of blood across the scalp. The purpose of
this was to make the lines clear through a layer of Betadine solution, which they now applied as a disinfectant.
When they were done, the blood continued to flow over the
skull like paint dripping on it from above.

"I hate beards," Benny said.

"What about it?" José said.

"Shit, he's worked on it a long time. Take it down to here
and leave the rest."

Benny drew a line with his finger just below the ear and
José used it as a guideline, shaving the edges of Charlie's

beard with a straight razor. He also shaved his eyebrows and went over the already shaven areas at the base of his skull.

Waiting for José to finish, Benny studied the angiograms again, outlining the tumor with his finger. Then he took a syringe from the instrument stand and injected Charlie's scalp with saline solution in half a dozen places, to reduce its vascularity in preparation for incision. Since each injection caused a swelling like a large hive, the scalp was pockmarked and disfigured. When Benny was done, it looked like the belly of a pregnant dog.

By now the urine bag beneath the table had begun to fill, and the steady beep of the oscilloscope could be heard, its beautiful jagged lines—readouts of pulse and blood pressure—marching across the screen above Charlie's feet. On the end of each line, for reasons I never could discover, was a five-pointed star which led it like a firefly. Because of the mannitol, which Carla had started a few minutes before, Charlie's pressure was low already, 100 over 65, but as the operation progressed and his bleeding became profuse, they would drop him at times as low as 65 over 45.

Everyone had read about a plane crash which had occurred the day before in South America, and conversation veered in that direction. Esther vowed she would never fly again, but Benny expressed an opinion I often heard from neurosurgeons, that the danger of flying was precisely what made it exciting.

"How many got killed?" José said.

"Eighty-five," said Esther.

"No," said Carla. "It was eighty-seven this morning on the radio."

Since Schreiber, his work load catching up to him, was sound asleep on a stool in a corner of the room, Carla was now in charge of Charlie's sleep. She was a tall, muscular woman with (as I discovered later when I saw her without her mask) an elegant face, hair cut short like a man's. In addition to her M.D., she had a Ph.D. in biophysics, and she had taken this residency because she hoped to do research in certain areas of neurochemistry. During the course of Charlie's procedure, she taught me more about anesthesiology than I had learned in all the time I'd been around the hospital.

Every thirty seconds Carla would make what she called eye rounds, checking vital signs by means of gauges on the anesthesia machine and listening—through earphones that trailed under the bed sheet and connected to a stethoscope—to Charlie's breathing (as done for him by the respirator) and heartbeat. It was her job to keep track of the drugs that dripped through the major I.V. from the bag that hung above the bed and make sure his intracranial pressure was kept low enough to prevent herniation but not so low that it exposed him to other problems. Since her work kept her close to his face, she was also, of all the people in the room, most aware of Charlie as a person. Leaning over now to adjust his bitelock, she glanced at his face and then at Millie, who was standing opposite her.

"Cute, isn't he?"

"Yeah," Millie said. "Nice guy, too."

The first incision, a quick slice with a scalpel along the forward line of the flap, was made by Benny at eight forty, and the scalp was peeled away from the muscle beneath it about fifteen minutes later. Three layers of tissue—scalp, muscle, and the membrane called the galea—had to be severed before bone was reached and drilling begun to prepare the area that Brockman, in his misguided attempt to assuage Mrs. White's anxiety, had called a trapdoor. Charlie's scalp was about a half inch and the bone about a quarter inch thick (it can be thicker or thinner at other points on the skull, and it also varies among individuals; two weeks earlier they had operated on a woman whose skull, according to Benny, was paper-thin). Altogether, it would take fifty-five minutes to complete the flap and expose the dura in preparation for Brockman's attack on the tumor.

Bleeding was heavy along the incision, and after the blood was suctioned and sponged, white plastic clips were installed to seal off the vessels. When the line of the flap had been incised, the tissue beneath it—called subaponeurotic—was sliced with a very sharp knife, then the flap was peeled back gently like the skin of an orange. There were many bleeding points on its underside, and as these were coagulated electrically, the now-familiar smell of burning skin filtered through the room.

"I'm losing a lot of blood," Benny said to Carla. "Can we take his pressure down?"

"A little," she said. "But not too much."

"How's your boyfriend?"

"Let's not talk about him."

"Why not?"

"I'd rather not say."

"Why not?"

"Leave me alone, Benny."

The flap was wrapped like a package, first with a mesh-like material, then with gauze, then clamped to the drape on its bottom side, just above Charlie's ear. Since the skull bone was covered with the galea, it was not yet visible, but now the galea was cut with a Bovie loop and pushed back gently with an instrument called a periosteal elevator. At the bottom of the flap, there was muscle to be got through in addition to galea, and this was cut with a scalpel.

"Call the Boss," Benny said. "Tell him thirty minutes."

When the bone was exposed, six large holes, about the size of those in a bowling ball, were drilled along the line of the flap. The instrument in this case was a nitrogen-powered, stainless-steel cylinder called a craniotome that looked a lot like a space gun and whined like a baby pig when activated. It took a half-inch bit for drilling and a slicing tool which made horizontal cuts. In their arsenal now for the last ten years, the craniotome's great feature was that, being air-powered, it responded negatively to pressure. The harder the tissue it encountered, the more power it generated. Thus, the drill bit turned with maximum speed through bone and stopped altogether when it met the soft tissue that lay beneath it.

Observing this procedure could increase one's respect for the human anatomy. The trait we call hardheadedness is not, it seems, entirely figurative. Benny had to get all his weight behind the craniotome to make it penetrate Charlie's skull. He leaned forward until his body was nearly thirty degrees off the vertical. The egglike shape of the skull is said to be inherently protective, distributing stress over the largest possible area, but the skullbone itself is tough as armor. Actually, it is armor. Monkey skulls—in what must be some of the more gruesome experiments scientists have devised—have been found capable of withstanding up to 1,500 pounds of pressure per square inch. Extrapolation of this information to the human head, which seems to be a bit harder than a monkey's, produces the estimate that a human skull can withstand accelerations of fifty to sixty times that of gravity on sudden impact of fifteen milliseconds' duration. In early vertebrates, armor covered the head and foreparts, but this added so much body weight that the animal more than lost in maneuverability what it gained in protection. The skull seems to be an evolutionary compromise with this problem, recognizing the fact that the brain requires a different sort of covering from the rest of the body. Certainly, as Benny was now demonstrating, it was not meant to be violated.

Shavings from the bone were kept in a paper cup on the instrument stand to plug the drill holes when the skull was reassembled. Each hole bled as drilled, and beeswax was applied as a sealer after it was suctioned and sponged.

When Benny was done with the craniotome, he took up a hand drill that looked exactly like a carpenter's, enlarged each hole, then clipped at the jagged edges with an instrument called a rongeur. Finally, when the holes were smoothed and coagulated, he set about connecting them.

There were various tools used for this, and that morning, since Charlie's skull was especially hard, Benny required them all. Using the craniotome with its cutting bit, he sawed out the line between the holes, angling the blade so that later, when the flap was replaced, the beveled edge would help secure it. Once again he had to lean into the drill with all his weight. Against heavy resistance from the bone, the saw moved very slowly, sometimes imperceptibly, sending trails of smoke into the room and generating so much heat that it required constant irrigation. Now, replacing the craniotome in its metal box, Benny threaded a flexible instrument called a dural protector between the holes and slid it back and forth several times to separate bone from the brain beneath it. He called for the rongeur again and clipped edges on the two holes closest to Charlie's ears, worked the space between them once again with the periosteal elevator, and finally, throwing the elevator onto the instrument stand, stood up—for the first time since his original incision—and surveyed his work.

"What's his pressure?"

"Ninety-five over seventy," Carla said.

"Can we take him down a point or two?"

"I'd rather not until we open the dura."

Benny shrugged his shoulders, rolled his head in a circle as if to stretch his neck, then looked up at Millie on the stand. "Chisels, please."

She handed him two stainless-steel instruments with blunt one-inch blades, slapping them between his thumb and forefinger. After working them first around the edges of the flap, Benny elevated it gently until he was certain it was coming off the dura, then grasped it with his fingers and lifted it clear. Now, for the first time, Charlie's brain was visible, framed by the flap and covered by the silky film of the dura like an embryo in its sack. Though the dura is protective and more opaque than transparent, one could discern quite clearly beneath it the interlacing of blood vessels on the surface of the brain and, just barely, the distinctive folds of the cortex.

The underside of the bone flap had grooves in it where the middle meningeal artery ran across the surface of the brain. This artery had been severed when Benny lifted the flap, and blood flowed heavily now until José suctioned it and Benny, using the cautery that passed current through the plate beneath Charlie's buttocks, sealed off the vessel. Now the flap was wrapped in moistened gauze, tied with rubber bands, and set up on the instrument stand, the dura irrigated, sponged, and dried, the drapes around the flap readjusted to prepare the neat, impersonal view which Brockman would require.

"What time is it?" Benny said.

"Nine twenty," Esther said.

"Anyone heard from the Boss?"

"He's on his way."

At this point in English operating rooms, orange juice is brought to the surgeons, delivered on sterile trays with straws that bend ingeniously to slip behind the surgeons' masks. No such civility in an American O.R.; Harvey Cushing's puritanical ghost is said to hover above them all. There was nothing for José and Benny to do while waiting for Brockman but put a towel over Charlie's brain and make a bit of small talk with the nurses.

About the time that Benny was calling for the chisels, Brockman had arrived in the locker room. He had dressed quickly and headed down the hall to scrub. His thoughts of Charlie? The last had occurred the night before, after evening rounds, when he'd paused a moment with Benny to review the angiograms and plan the flap. Touching his own head on the crown, just to the right of the midline, he'd said, "Get me down here, all right?" Benny had nodded, and that was it. This morning he'd not once glanced in Charlie's direction.

In the washroom he met a heart surgeon named Chester Freed, and leaning over the sink they talked about Vienna. Freed was on his way there for a conference, and Brockman, who had been in Europe two months before, had a restaurant he wanted Freed to try.

"Stopping in Paris?"

"No, I'm going through Rome to see my daughter."

As always Brockman took a scrub sponge into the O.R. and continued to wash, dripping suds on the floor, while he inspected the flap that Benny had turned.

"Looks good," he said. "Jesus, Benny, you're getting better all the time."

He stood with his back to Millie while she dressed him, examined the angiograms while she pulled on his gloves, and finally stepped up between José and Benny and probed the dura with his finger. His face was eight to ten inches from Charlie's brain.

"Lower the table a couple of inches, please."

"I'm sorry, sir," Esther said. "I thought you wanted it—"

"That wasn't a criticism. Just lower the table."

The motor in the table honked like an auto horn, and Charlie's head moved down until it offered a better angle.

"What's his pressure?"

"Ninety-five over seventy," Carla said.

Stretching his hand toward Millie, Brockman requested Malis scissors and then quickly opened the dura. Taut and resilient, it snapped out of the way, and the brain pushed through the opening like a tiny fist. Fifteen years ago, this was a dangerous moment in neurosurgery, because brains expanded drastically and often herniated when the dura

was opened, but nowadays, with steroids to control intracranial pressure, the swelling was not problematic.

It was nine thirty-five. After making a small incision, the
Boss inserted a strip of Cottonoid between the dura and
the brain and then continued cutting, using the Cottonoid
as a protective buffer, sliding it along as the incision progressed. In time he cut out a piece of dura which more or
less followed the flap, taking care not to use the cautery
too much, since it caused contraction in the dura that
might make it too tight to close. Finally, the dural flap was
raised as the bone and muscle had been raised before it,
wrapped in moistened gauze, and clamped out of the way.
In all its convolution, oyster-gray and pink on its surface
and almost black at the folds, the cortex was visible at last.
It was nine forty-five.

At the bottom of the exposure lay the tumor. Encap-
sulated like all meningiomas, it was striated with blood
vessels like the brain around it but (unlike Billy Eggleston's tumor) still sharply distinct from it, darker and
smoother, clearly alien but inoffensive somehow, certainly
anticlimactic. Hard to believe that this walnut-sized collection of cells which the brain had produced of its own accord
had dropped Charlie to the floor more than four weeks ago
when he stood up from his desk.

One of the crucial variables with parasagittal meningiomas (since they originate in the lining of the brain) is
whether they've invaded the transparent membrane called
the arachnoid which lies beneath the dura. If so, a layer of
brain must be removed along with the tumor, and the
chance of deficit in the aftermath of surgery is greatly
enhanced. Seeking this information, Brockman probed the
arachnoid with a forceps, then edged his retractor around
the mass—bending it so that it followed the tumor's
contours—to determine as much as he could about its
depth. When a good view had been exposed, he called
for the microscope and the videotape, and a moment

later Charlie's brain made its first appearance on television.

"Okay," said the Boss. "We're looking at this man's motor strip. That's leg and that's arm. That's tongue. Since the tumor gave him a leg seizure, we know it's growing to the falx. The arachnoid is involved, even some of the dura, I think, but there's no reason from what I see that we shouldn't get it all."

It seemed to me that Charlie's chances had taken a sudden nose dive, but I was wrong. As Benny explained later, the region in which the arachnoid and dura were involved was not near enough to vital centers to endanger his motor function. Though another surgeon might have been intimidated by a tumor so invasive, Brockman had done so many over the years that he handled it with no timidity at all.

The first target with meningiomas is their blood supply. Since they're highly vascular tumors, they can hemorrhage if entered directly, but once their principal sources have been tied off, they can be manageable, even tame. In search of the feeding vessels, Brockman worked his way around the tumor, using his retractor first and then Cottonoid, coagulating with a hyphercator when vessels were small, a Bovie forceps when they were large. Once or twice, in what seemed to me an ingenious improvisation (I found out later it was common), he gripped his suction tube with his coagulating forceps so that he sent current down the barrel of the tube and coagulated as he drew off the loose tissue and blood that he'd produced.

With all that cutting they were using the suction tube a lot, and, as sometimes happens, this led to misadventure. Suddenly a piece of normal brain got caught up and sucked —*whoosh!*—up the tube, gone forever into the central garbage receptacle that served the suction tubes in all operating rooms on the floor. I had seen this happen before, though not with crucial tissue (as we've seen, they avoided

vital regions if they could). This time, with Brockman working in such proximity to Charlie's motor strip, I thought
he'd sucked an arm or leg right up the tube. As it turned
out, I was wrong again. The normal tissue came from the
posterior side of the tumor, far from anything crucial, and
the brain that disappeared would not be missed. To say the
least, Brockman took its departure in stride.

"Shit," he said. "There go the music lessons."

Everyone in the room cracked up, Benny grunting behind his mask and Millie convulsing on the stand, but the
pleasure was short-lived because José got his suction tube
entangled with the Boss's.

"Hey, José, you sleeping? Come on! Move it out of the
way! Why are you so timid? Three months we've worked
together and you're acting like a schoolboy."

By ten o'clock Brockman had the tumor ligated and separated (with Cottonoid) from the brain around it. To ele-
vate or, as the surgeons say, mobilize the tumor, he sewed
several sutures to it and then attached them to clamps,
drawing them taut and lifting the tumor a bit from its
cavity. His anger had settled, and the conversation at the
table became polite and friendly, almost intimate.

"Speech problem, you think?" José asked.

"I doubt it," Brockman replied. "Bayonet, please."

"Irrigation," Benny said.

"Oh, that's pretty, isn't it?" Brockman said. "Make a
sharper bend in your retractor, Benny. Yes, that's it.
That's very nice. No, no. You take the retractor, José, and
give me the sucker. When it's bleeding, I've got to control
it myself."

When things were quiet like this, the sounds of the O.R.
were musical and hypnotic. The sizzle of the cautery, the
flutelike beep of the oscilloscope, the sighs of the respirator, the conversation, the suction, the clink of instruments
against each other like knives and forks at the dinner table
—it was all repetitive, monotonous, constant in its rhythm

as a fugue. If you listened with enough detachment, all of it merged in a sweet continuum that might have been made on a synthesizer.

Brockman came now upon the large draining vessel called the sagittal sinus, which he'd mentioned to Charlie in their first interview. In certain cases parasagittal meningiomas invade crucial areas of this sinus, and if it is transected during surgery, the result can be coma or quadriplegia. (As Brockman had pointed out to Charlie, the danger was actually less if the tumor was blocking the sinus entirely.) In Charlie's case, as it turned out, the sinus vein was not invaded, but—equally dangerous—it blocked the only angle by which the tumor could be approached.

When the Boss had a good view of the sinus, he called for the videotape again and pointed (with his forceps) to a vein which was actually connected to the sinus. "We must preserve this vein at any cost. It's draining the motor strip into the sinus."

Continuing the tape, since this was essential technique for students, he slipped Cottonoid behind and in front of the vein, trying to isolate and secure it, but a moment later it slipped forward anyway, and a bit of hysteria ensued.

"Shit! Watch out! Get the fuck outa there, Benny! Move it! Move it! How many times I got to tell you, don't cross over me when I've got cutting instruments in my hand."

As it turned out, the problem was a piece of dura which had been invaded by tumor and was itself pulling on the vein. Once they amputated it and slipped more Cottonoid between the vein and the adjoining tissue, everything was under control. As for the hysteria, which was rarely thus captured on the videotape, it was the highlight of Friday conference.

By ten fifteen they were extracting tumor.

"We could deliver it all in spectacular fashion for the tape," Brockman said, "but it's a helluva lot better for this guy to gut it and take it piecemeal."

Using a scalpel first and then a copper spoon, he broke through the tumor's capsule and dug it out in small, bloody slivers, which he placed in the specimen glass on the instrument stand. The inside of the tumor looked a lot like Cream of Wheat. Once gutted, its walls collapsed, and the difficult points at which it was connected to brain became accessible. By ten forty, half the tumor was in the specimen glass and the rest had snaked away through the suction tube. The Boss was packing the empty cavity with Gelfoam, a Styrofoam-like material that expands when it's wet and contracts as it dries, promoting coagulation in the areas beneath it. A few minutes later, he said, "All right, let's get the hell out of there."

By the time he had showered and dressed and made his way to the ninth floor where, to use his words for it, he played a bit of God for Mrs. White and Roberta, Charlie was almost reassembled.

Closing was tedious and time-consuming, more hazardous in certain ways than opening. The danger of clots or postoperative bleeding was not a small one, and there were no miraculous instruments to protect against it. No oscilloscope recorded a vein left open, no lights blinked if a flap were improperly sealed. As usual, tension had diminished with the Boss's departure, but, relaxed though the mood became, there was no interruption of the burden or the concentration it required. ("The worst part of a party," Benny said. "Cleaning up when it's over.") José and Benny had seen too many mistakes to let that happen, too much postsurgical hemorrhage after perfectly successful operations, too many patients returning like unicorns, their bone flaps infected and disfigured like Rosie Galindez's.

The Boss had closed the dura before he left and sewn a patch called Silastic over the area he had amputated. Now Benny and José set about reconstructing the rest of Charlie's skull, starting with the bone.

When the dura was cleaned and dried, a plastic tube, beginning at the highest point on the skull, was laid across it to act as a siphon, a gravity-fed drain to draw off excess fluid. Tiny, pinlike holes were drilled (with the craniotome) in the bone flap and used to wire the flap to the skull, and stainless-steel sutures, threaded through these holes, were twisted together and stuffed in nearby burr holes, there to remain—like the Silastic patch—for the rest of Charlie's life. They were moving along, and Benny was whistling behind his mask.

"I hear you're taking us to lunch," Millie said.

"You kidding?" Benny said. "I've got an aneurysm this afternoon."

"What did I tell you, Esther?"

"They're too cheap," Esther said. "The ENT people, they take us all the time. I never yet got a meal from a neurosurgeon."

"We got no heart, that's our trouble," José said. "We're all locked up in our heads."

Burr holes were filled first with Gelfoam and then with the bone shavings that had been collected during the original drilling. The bone was inspected carefully for bleeding spots, and once it was attached, the inner surface of the muscle above it was heavily cauterized, then sutured to the muscle on the skull surrounding it. One small opening was left in the flap for the drain, which was pushed through a special hole (called a stab wound) made especially for it behind Charlie's ear. The drain would remain in place, attached to Charlie's bandage like a feather on a cap, for thirty-six hours, and then, if his intracranial pressure was satisfactory, they'd remove it and sew up the wound. The opening in the bone—actually one of the burr holes—was not considered problematic.

Esther was counting sponges aloud—"Ninety-one, ninety-two, ninety-three"—tying them in packages of a hundred for disposal. During an operation like this they could go through two, three, or even four such packages. "What are you doing tonight?" she asked Millie.

"I don't know. Maybe I'll kill myself."

"Well, do me a favor," Benny said. "Don't shoot yourself in the head. I've got a busy schedule tomorrow."

With the under layer of flap in place, they had continued to the muscle and periosteum. Now they were restoring the scalp, and there was a lot of sewing to be done. Unlike their orthopedic colleagues, they couldn't use a staple gun, so each stitch was personal and meticulous handiwork, inserted by hand, knotted by hand, loose ends clipped by hand. Sutures were made of fine silk material (other specialties have opted for synthetics, but not the neurosurgeons) which had been threaded—in tiny U-shaped needles —by the manufacturer. Esther removed them one by one from their packages, installed them in a special instrument, and passed the instrument to Benny, who pushed the needle through the edges he meant to knit, tied the knot, then passed it to José, who clipped the loose ends. The needle, like the sponges and syringes and Cottonoid, was thrown away. By the time they were done, they had taken more than one hundred and fifty stitches in Charlie's scalp.

They were standing in a pool of blood at least half an inch deep, the floor around them littered with miscellaneous junk—gauzes and sponges and strips of Cottonoid. Esther and Millie ran a pretty tight ship, but there was no way to keep ahead of the mess, especially when they were working on the scalp. The region between the scalp and the galea is highly vascular, and they did not like to coagulate it too much because they wanted it to heal inconspicuously, and that requires maximum blood supply. Thus, heavy bleeding ensued when the clips which had held the scalp and galea together were removed, and there was nothing to stop it but sponges and sutures. It wasn't dangerous, but it certainly inflated the pool at their feet.

By noon Charlie's scalp was in place. Since the drapes were not yet removed, one could not see the curvature of his skull or detect any human connotation in the object on the table, but if one tried very hard, vague memories stirred of the man who had lifted himself onto the table almost five hours before. To me, Charlie was a friend I'd not seen for years but expected to meet soon again.

Apropos of nothing, Esther said, "In my opinion, this is the most boring room on the floor. Cut and suck, cut and suck. All you do is cut and suck."

"Umm," Benny said, "that sounds pretty good to me."

When the last suture was in, when the scalp was cleaned and irrigated and the drain plugged into the bulblike receptacle which would store the fluid it collected, Benny wiped the skull once more with a moistened sponge and said, "All right, Carla, bring him up."

Carla closed off the halothane and pancuronium (injecting a drug called antiacetylcholinesterase to counteract the pancuronium), and almost at once Charlie was breathing for himself. It was twelve fifteen. While Benny wrapped his bandage (one of the few reasons for pain in neurosurgery is a bandage incorrectly fitted), José peeled away the drapes, and piece by piece, first an ear and a bit of cheek and then a corner of the mouth, Charlie's face reappeared. There was an instant, only an instant, when the brain I'd just seen and the face I saw now were joined in my mind, but such interrelationships, as I've noted, were not exactly manageable, not, it seemed to me, the normal inclination of one's mind. After a moment, appropriate amnesia resumed, and the illusion of the head in all its glory was revived. Charlie was of a piece, his identity defined by his appearance, which the surgeons, it seemed to me, had fabricated like magicians.

"I'm going to lunch," Benny said, stripping off his gloves.

"Take me," Esther said.

"I've seen enough of you."

Terry Schreiber, wide awake now, leaned over Charlie. There was blood under his eye patches, and his mouth was twisted out of all recognition by the bitelock and the tracheal tube. Only a corpse could be more devoid of color.

"What's his name?" Terry said.

"Charlie," Esther said.

"Charlie? Charlie! Charlie! Wake up! Surgery is over! Everything is fine! Wake up, Charlie!"

Schreiber continued to holler like this for ten or fifteen seconds while Carla removed the tracheal tube and the bitelock and quickly suctioned Charlie's throat with another instrument, to draw off mucus that had collected during surgery. When she withdrew the tube, his tongue emerged—a voluntary movement at last, initiated by that part of his brain which had just recently been the Boss's target—and made a great sweep across his lips.

"Hunhh," he whispered. "Hunhh."

"Don't cough!" Schreiber cried. "Don't move those arms!"

José leaned over his face. "I'm going to untape your eyes now, Charlie."

Charlie's lids fluttered but did not open. Like the rest of his face, they appeared to be devoid of energy. Time and again he licked his lips, but no other muscles stirred.

Esther went out to the hall for his bed, and José removed the sheet that had covered him during surgery. Since the catheter in his penis would remain in place for the next couple of days, the urine bag was piled on his naked belly to be transferred along with him to the recovery room and, later today, the I.C.U. on the ninth floor. The flap drain, of course, was attached to his bandaged head, and the principal I.V. line, since steroids would be continued, remained on the stand above him.

When Esther had returned with his bed, she and Millie each took a leg and Schreiber grabbed him by the shoul-

ders, and crying "One, two, three!" they slid him off the
operating table to the place where he'd begun his day.
Then they wrapped him in a clean sheet, shifted his I.V.
line to the stand above the bed, and rolled him out and
down the hall, through the swinging doors, past the elevators, past the aneurysm patient that Benny would do this
afternoon.

Just before they took him into the recovery room,
Charlie opened his eyes briefly and saw me at the end of
his bed.

"How you doing?" I asked.

"Tired," he said. "Guess pretty tired."

By three that afternoon he was in the I.C.U., and by
seven that evening he was talking to his mother while
Roberta, as promised, held a microphone close to his
mouth. Two days later, he was released from the I.C.U.
and returned to a regular room on the ward. By then it had
been determined that there was no deficit, either in his leg
or in his tongue. He would need no radiation or chemotherapy because the tumor, as Brockman had predicted, had
turned out benign, but he would be on Dilantin and phenobarbital for five years at least, to protect him from seizures, and like George Tinker he would have to consider
himself, for the rest of his life, prone to meningioma.

His skin healed in a week, muscle and bone in seventy
days. According to Brockman, all traces of surgery were
gone from his brain within a year. Nothing was said or
postulated about its traces in his mind, but then, as they
say, nothing was done to his mind anyway.

Epilogue

Nineteen months after surgery, Charlie White was functioning, if anything, better than before. A recent CAT-scan had shown no sign of recurring meningioma, and after reading it, Brockman had discontinued his phenobarbital (because of which he had been sleeping twelve to fourteen hours a day) and taken him down to three Dilantins, the daily dose he'd probably maintain as long as he lived.

Looking back, he called neurosurgery "a thrill" and "a voyage into the unknown." The worst part of it had been the depression he'd entered upon return from the hospital, three months of no meaning and absolute boredom with excitements of the past. Gradually he had eased himself back into an everyday existence that was more or less oblivious to death, but he still believed that surgery had left him "more in touch" and "less concerned with petty things." "When I see someone upset with something insignificant, like missing a bus or staining a shirt, I can't believe my eyes."

He was teaching again (his students more challenging and responsive than in his previous job), and he had an idea for a book about the movies. The book he'd planned on neurosurgery was long forgotten. Unlike many surgical patients, he could remember his experience in the hospital, but everything he'd written about it had been, in his opinion, sentimental and banal. Though the scar beneath his now-thick head of hair was proof that neurosurgery had happened to him, he often thought of it as of a dream. And for all the clarity of his recollection, he was not inclined to speak of neurosurgery, not terribly interested in seeing those (like me) who reminded him where he'd been.

None of that, of course, had anything to do with Brockman. What mattered to the Boss was the scan and the absence of neurological deficit. Charlie would visit once a year, phone if anything strange occurred, and, like most postsurgical patients, have annual CAT-scans, but otherwise it was taken for granted that he was on his own.

Since leaving the hospital, Charlie had phoned Brockman once, eight months after surgery, when he had developed the queasy sense that water was dripping on his head. Occasionally, too, he heard a sound "like cracking knuckles" whenever he raised his eyebrows. Brockman listened and dismissed him: "Doesn't mean a thing to me." It was part of Charlie's history but not his neurosurgical file that, not completely satisfied with Brockman's response, he'd then sought out a faith healer, who had cupped her hands above his incision and—after listening in for a moment on the astral plane—confirmed his neurological health. "Don't worry," she said. "There's nothing wrong with your brain."

George Tinker was doing all right too. He walked with a limp, but his scan, like Charlie's, was clear, and during the summer he'd developed a passion for swimming that, for the first time since his return from Canada, had given him a sense of physical well-being. With the aid of a brace, he walked without a cane, and now that he had a left-foot accelerator, he drove himself alone wherever he wanted to go. Fourteen months after surgery, he flew to the West

Coast on business, his first such trip in twenty-six months. Considering his past experience, the voyage was nothing less than heroic, but he spoke of it characteristically: "What the hell, I like to see new places."

He was doing free-lance public relations work, but money was a problem. Six months before, he'd sent out 400 résumés and received one response. During the course of that interview, he had spoken of his medical history ("You might as well know that there's this problem, and I can't tell if it's gonna come back or not . . . all I can say is I've done my job except for three times"), and a polite rejection had arrived two weeks later.

His greatest problem was not directly related to neurosurgery. Soon after he'd returned to free-lance work, his wife, who'd borne the brunt of his illness for seventeen years, had begun to disintegrate emotionally. During the past six months, she had been virtually incapacitated. There were physical symptoms—anemia, rectal bleeding, colon irritation—and it was entirely possible, of course, that her problem had nothing to do with his, but the timing of her illness seemed remarkable to both of them. In fact, she dated her depression from the time George had obtained his left-foot accelerator and, with it, the freedom to travel without her help. They were not the first family I'd met who had experienced this reversal. There is nothing like nursing physical illness for helping the nurse deny psychological problems, no panic like that which descends when the physical illness improves.

Mary Ellen Bench was doing so well that Kenneth Beck called her an "advertisement for neurosurgery." This child whose language centers had been so recently endangered was now an excellent student at school. Unless one searched very carefully beneath her hair, one could not differentiate her from her classmates. What Beck would never forget about her case was the second opinion her family had almost accepted, the prominent neurosurgeon who had assured them that Mary Ellen's tumor was inoperable: no way to approach it without leaving her permanently brain damaged. Beck considered Mary Ellen's case perfect evidence to support the argument for the centralization of neurosurgical facilities. "That guy was no fool. He just hadn't seen enough of her kind of lesion to know what he was talking about."

More good news, briefly. Rosie Galindez had completely recovered, her forehead returned to its normal curvature. Both Dr. Chardan and Mr. Sedgwick were still alive and moving about without assistance. Allan Benjamin had eye trouble and a bit of facial paralysis, but his scan was clear and his mind no more (or less) obsessive than before. Marvin Welsh, though still of course retarded and hemiplegic, had suffered no seizures since his hemispherectomy. Victor Alfredo was aphasic, but there was no giant aneurysm in his head. For better or worse, he could expect to live out his life without further problems.

Bad news? Sister Callahan died three months after her encounter with Tony Kirtz, and Tony himself never left the hospital; a heart attack killed him two days after their meeting in the hall. Raymond Dreyer, aphasia undiminished, had lived six months after surgery and died peacefully in his sleep.

Billy Eggleston was not so lucky. Surgery gave him six good months, but he paid for them with almost a year of nightmare. In the fall, after his operation the previous spring, he was swimming, riding his bike, and attending school. His parents considered him perfectly healthy. By November, his headaches had returned and with them, now, double vision and lethargy. His scan revealed a tumor that no one considered operable, but his parents pleaded with Beck (whom Brockman had now assigned to Billy's case) to have a go at it. Billy had his second craniotomy in early December, and he was never functional again. The operation left him paralyzed on his right side and, though responsive to questions, offering nothing in the way of spontaneous conversation. Against Beck's advice, he was given chemotherapy. In June of the following year, a scan revealed a tumor 53mm wide that had invaded Billy's corpus callosum and both hemispheres of his brain. Once again the parents pleaded and once again Beck relented. Billy had a third craniotomy in early July and received still another course of chemotherapy. On October 20, Beck received the following note from the neurologist who'd been treating Billy at his hometown in Pennsylvania:

> Dear Ken:
>
> Shortly after our telephone conversations yesterday, Billy Eggleston stopped breathing. I reinstituted ventricular drainage but to no avail. His mother insisted we begin mechanical ventilation. He expired 12 hours later.
>
> Best wishes to you and Susan from Nancy and me.

That same month saw the publication, six months after his death, of the book that Peter Fleischman had worked on for nearly twelve years before brain damage forced him to put it down. It was a large, ambitious statement, well received by his professional colleagues, little noticed by anyone else. Like most psychoanalytic tracts, it was built on a limitless faith in the ability of mind to conquer matter, the consummate power of "understanding" in the treatment of "mental" problems. It was Fleischman's belief that one was "responsible" for his anxiety and his conflict and that anyone who "accepted" this responsibility would be able to discern the roots of his pain and dissolve it. Speaking of a patient who'd developed breast cancer, for example, he postulated a causal connection between the malignancy and the patient's feelings toward her mother's death, concluding, "This patient, like many others, suggested to me the powerful relationship between psychic factors and malignancy, though they have yet to be scientifically verified."

No one would ever know, of course, whether his own malignancy had induced him to strengthen or reverse such opinion, or whether, for that matter, his tumor had not been present—and influential—in his brain when he wrote it down.

NOTES

Chapter 1: Trapdoor

PAGE

21. ... *a recent study*. "A Summary Report of the Study of Surgical Services in the United States," sponsored by the American College of Surgeons and the American Surgical Association, 1975.

Chapter 2: The Perfect Tension

34. Both Kurt Goldstein and A. R. Luria have written extensively on the subject of brain damage. See especially Goldstein's *Human Nature* (New York: Schocken, 1963) and Luria's *The Man with the Shattered World* (New York: Basic Books, 1972); also, on brain damage in general, Howard Gardner's *The Shattered Mind* (New York: Knopf, 1975).

Chapter 3: A Certain Frame of Mind

81. *The Montreal procedure*. Exquisite photos of brains involved may be found in *Speech and Brain Mechanisms* by Wilder Penfield and Lamar Roberts (Princeton, N.J.: Princeton University Press, 1959).

81. *"more psychical."* Wilder Penfield's *The Mystery of Mind* (Princeton, N.J.: Princeton University Press, 1975), p. 52.

82. "*doubling of awareness.*" Ibid., p. 55.

82. "*the content of consciousness.*" Ibid.

82. *The jury remained out.* . . . There is of course no end to the speculation that continues in this area. Readers who wish to explore it further might begin with *The Self and Its Brain* by Karl Popper and John Eccles (Berlin, London and New York: Springer International, 1977).

Chapter 4: Managing Power

93. On microsurgical techniques, see: "Microvascular Surgery for Stroke" by Jack M. Fein, *Scientific American*, April 1978.

97. On the reticular formation: *The Conscious Brain* by Steven Rose (New York: Vintage, 1976), p. 295.

102. On split-brain patients: "The Great Cerebral Commissure" by Roger Sperry, in *The Biological Bases of Behavior*, ed. by N. R. Chalmers, R. Crawley, and S.P.R. Rose (New York: Harper & Row, 1971).

Chapter 5: Origins

110. Much of this chapter owes a very large debt to two books in particular: *The Conscious Brain* by Steven Rose (cited in the notes for chapter 4) and *The Human Brain* by Isaac Asimov (New York: New American Library, 1963). There is a tremendous literature in this field, but I have found these two works to be the most literate and accessible. They are enthusiastically recommended to anyone who wishes to read further.

118. . . . *conflict between the "new" brain and the "old."*Arthur Koestler's *The Ghost in the Machine* (New York: Macmillan, 1968).

118. For an excellent discussion of simplistic neuropsychology, see "What We Know (and Don't Know) About the Two Halves of the Brain" by Howard Gardner, *Harvard Magazine*, March–April 1978.

123. Cushing's arrival on the scene: E. H. Thomson, *Harvey Cushing* (New York: Schuman, 1950).

125. On the operating microscope: Holmgren used a binocular microscope, which afforded three-dimensional viewing. The principal modification for neurosurgery was a system by which direct illumi-

nation was provided through the same optical system which mag- nifies the operating field. See article by Fein cited in the notes for chapter 4.

126. *Techniques in stereotaxis*: These were developed primarily by H. T. Wycis and E. A. Spiegel and modernized by (among others) I. S. Cooper in New York and J. Talairach in France. For medical reference see Wycis and Spiegel's *Stereo-Encephalotomy* (New York: Grune & Stratton, 1962); for the general reader, see Cooper's *The Victim Is Always the Same* (New York: Harper & Row, 1973).

126. *... the political and moral problems of psychosurgery*: In the late 1930s and early 1940s, lobotomies were often performed in a doc- tor's office, sometimes with tools that weren't much more sophisticated than ice picks. For particularly graphic descriptions of these proce- dures, see Walter J. Freeman and James W. Watts, *Psychosurgery* (Springfield, Ill.: Charles C Thomas, 1942).

Although prefrontal lobotomy has fallen into disfavor, stereotaxis opens up another area in which neurosurgeons can approach psycholog- ical problems, and it is here that delicate political issues will arise. In the United States, there seems to be a great deal of inhibition in this area, but it is being explored in other countries with enthusiasm. A recent anthology—*Psychosurgery*, edited by E. Hitchcock, L. Laitinen, and K. Vaernet (Springfield, Ill.: Charles C Thomas, 1972)—lists chap- ters describing the surgical treatment of the following "diseases": mood disturbance, obsessive syndromes, aggression, violence, compul- siveness, restless behavior, and pedophilic homosexuality and "other sexual deviations."

Chapter 6: One Lovely Doctor

151. "*The enterprise of biomedical research. ...*" Lewis Thomas, *Science*, vol. 200 (June 30, 1978), p. 1459.

162. "*It is interesting. ...*" Eric J. Cassell, *The Healer's Art* (Phila- delphia: Lippincott, 1976), p. 142.

Chapter 7: A Bounty of Mementos

169. For a remarkable, if harrowing, description of encephalitis, see *Awakening* by Oliver Sacks (New York: Random, 1976).

Chapter 8: Inappropriate Smiles

211. Hughlings Jackson is quoted in "Complementarity as a Rule in Psychological Research: Jackson, Freud and the Mind-Body Problem," by Henry Edelheit, *International Journal of Psychoanalysis*, vol. 57, p. 23 (1976).

213. *"When you make the two one. . . ."* The Gospel According to Thomas. Coptic text established and translated by A. Guillaumont. Henri-Charles Peuch, Gilles Quispel, Walter Till, and Yassah Abd. Al Masih (New York: Harper & Row, 1959), p. 17.

214. *"Form is emptiness. . . ."* Prajna-Parmita-hridaya Sutra, in F. M. Muller, ed., *Sacred Books of the East*, vol. XLIX, *Buddhist Mahayana Sutras*.

Chapter 9: The Music Lessons

253. On the skull's resilience, see D. F. Cavness and A. E. Walker, *Head Injury* (Philadelphia: Lippincott, 1966).

253. *. . . an evolutionary compromise.* Asimov (op. cit. in notes for chapter 5), p. 145.